BestMasters

Springer awards „BestMasters" to the best master's theses which have been completed at renowned universities in Germany, Austria, and Switzerland. The studies received highest marks and were recommended for publication by supervisors. They address current issues from various fields of research in natural sciences, psychology, technology, and economics.The series addresses practitioners as well as scientists and, in particular, offers guidance for early stage researchers.

Elena Hitzel

Effects of Peripheral Vision on Eye Movements

A Virtual Reality Study on Gaze Allocation in Naturalistic Tasks

With a foreword by Prof. Karl R. Gegenfurtner, Ph.D.

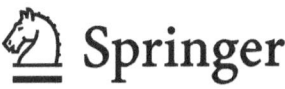 Springer

Elena Hitzel
Münzenberg, Germany

OnlinePLUS Material zu diesem Buch finden Sie auf
http://www.springer.de/ 978-3-658-08465-3

BestMasters
ISBN 978-3-658-08465-3   ISBN 978-3-658-08466-0 (eBook)
DOI 10.1007/978-3-658-08466-0

Library of Congress Control Number: 2014958972

Springer

Printed on acid-free paper

Springer is a brand of Springer Fachmedien Wiesbaden
Springer Fachmedien Wiesbaden is part of Springer Science+Business Media
(www.springer.com)

Geleitwort

Blickbewegungen spielen eine enorm wichtige Rolle bei der Informationsaufnahme aus unserer Umwelt. Nur in einem kleinen Bereich des Gesichtsfelds, so groß wie der Daumennagel auf Armlänge, erreichen wir die optimale Sehschärfe. Gerade für die Steuerung von Bewegungen ist diese präzise Information dringlich von Nöten. Leider wurden Blickbewegungen bislang vornehmlich in ganz einfachen Konfigurationen untersucht, bei denen der Blick zum Beispiel auf einen peripher dargebotenen Punkt gerichtet werden muss.

Die Master-Arbeit von Elena Hitzel beschreitet hier einen gänzlich neuen innovativen Ansatz. In einer Virtuellen Umwelt gingen die Probanden durch einen Raum und hatten dabei die Aufgabe, bestimmte Objekte einzusammeln und andere zu vermeiden. Dabei wurde der Einfluss von zusätzlichen, peripher dargebotenen, Objekten auf die Blickposition bestimmt. Tatsächlich waren die Blickpositionen auf dem fixierten Objekt in Richtung des benachbarten Objekts verschoben. Dieser Effekt war stärker ausgeprägt, wenn das benachbarte Objekt aufgabenrelevant war. Dies legt nahe, dass die Auswahl von Fixationspositionen nicht nur durch die aktuelle Aufgabe und das aktuell fixierte Objekt bestimmt wird, sondern mehrere Objekte und Aufgaben gleichzeitig die Fixationsposition beeinflussen können.

Die Arbeit von Frau Hitzel wurden im Rahmen einer Kollaboration mit Prof. Mary Hayhoe und Prof. Dana Ballard an der University of Texas at Austin (Texas, USA) durchgeführt, die als Pioniere der Erforschung menschlicher Wahrnehmung in virtuellen Welten gelten.

Obwohl es sich hier natürlich in erster Linie um Grundlagenforschung handelt, ergeben sich wichtige Aspekte für verschiedene Anwendungsfelder, vor allem für die Gestaltung der Darbietung von Information im peripheren Gesichtsfeld.

Prof. Karl R. Gegenfurtner, Ph.D.

Gießen im Oktober 2014

Institutsprofil

Die Psychologie in Giessen kann auf eine lange Tradition verweisen. So wurde 1904 die Deutsche Gesellschaft für Experimentelle Psychologie, aus der später die Deutsche Gesellschaft für Psychologie hervorging, in Giessen gegründet. Von 1911 bis 1927 war Kurt Koffka, Mitbegründer der Gestaltpsychologie, in Giessen tätig. In neuerer Zeit zeichnet sich die Giessener Psychologie als forschungsstark aus, was sich in vielen Rankings widerspiegelt, vor allem auch im Förder-Ranking der Deutschen Forschungsgemeinschaft. Mit drei Professuren nimmt die Abteilung Allgemeine Psychologie eine zentrale Stellung ein. Die Abteilung um Katja Fiehler, Roland Fleming und Karl Gegenfurtner genießt inzwischen weltweites Renommee durch hervorragende und innovative Arbeit im Bereich der visuellen Wahrnehmung und visuell gesteuerter Handlung. So steht die Abteilung an der Spitze des von der DFG geförderten Sonderforschungsbereichs „Kardinale Mechanismen der Wahrnehmung", eines von der DFG geförderten internationalen Graduierten-kollegs „The brain in action" mit Partnern aus Kanada, und eines von der EU finanzierten Research Training Network zur Wahrnehmung von Oberflächen.

Contents

Abstracts

English

Gaze is a reliable indicator of visual attention in a variety of everyday situations. Thus far, some models of top-down driven gaze allocation, such as the model suggested by Sprague, Ballard, and Robinson (2007), predict humans' visuomotor behavior assuming that visual information is gathered from only one object at a time.

Contrary to this simplifying premise are the findings that visual input from the periphery influences gaze deployment, as shown for instance by the visual center of gravity effect (Findlay, 1982; Vishwanath & Kowler, 2003).

The interaction of these two ideas, namely the useful exploitation of peripheral information in natural vision remained largely unexplored. Therefore, the present study pursues the idea that people show a gaze bias towards non-fixated neighboring objects in terms of a compromise between foveal and peripheral information gain.

Using Virtual Reality software, eye movements were recorded through eye tracking devices as subjects ($N=12$) were walking through a virtual environment gathering targets and/or avoiding obstacles.

As hypothesized, the data analysis showed that fixations biased towards a neighboring object tend to be made more frequently than fixations biased in the opposite direction, independent of object configuration and task. Additionally, this effect was even more distinct when the neighboring object was relevant to the current task, but only significantly increased when subjects were doing two tasks at once.

In conclusion, these results indicate that peripheral information influences gaze allocation in naturalistic tasks. Since this gaze bias additionally depends on task-relevance of the neighboring object and by association on reward, it can be interpreted as a useful gaze strategy. Hence, the exclusive role of foveal vision in models of gaze behavior should be reconsidered.

German

Wohin eine Person schaut, gilt in vielen alltäglichen Situationen als zuverlässiger Indikator dafür, worauf sie gerade ihre visuelle Aufmerksamkeit richtet.

Einige Modelle, die die Rolle von sogenannten ,top-down' Prozessen in der Steuerung natürlicher Augenbewegungen betonen, wie beispielsweise das von Sprague, Ballard und Robinson (2007), treffen Vorhersagen bezüglich der visuomotorischen Steuerung unter der Prämisse, dass zu jedem Zeitpunkt nur die visuelle Information eines einzelnen Objektes herangezogen werden kann.

Dieser vereinfachenden Annahme entgegen, stehen Befunde, wie etwa der sogenannte visuelle ,Center of Gravity'-Effekt (z.B. Findlay, 1982; Vishwanath & Kowler, 2003), die zeigen, dass visuelle Informationen aus dem peripheren Gesichtsfeld Blickbewegungen beeinflussen können.

Das Zusammenspiel dieser beiden Ideen, nämlich die sinnvolle Nutzung peripherer Informationen unter natürlichen Bedingungen, blieb bislang weitgehend unerforscht. Daher verfolgt die vorliegende Studie die Annahme, dass Personen, im Sinne eines Kompromisses zwischen fovealem und peripherem Informationsgewinn, eine Verschiebung der Blickposition in Richtung anderer nicht-fixierter Objekte zeigen.

Mit Hilfe einer Software zur Erstellung einer virtuellen Realität wurden Augenbewegungen mittels Eye-Tracker aufgezeichnet während die Versuchs-teilnehmer (N = 12) durch einen virtuellen Raum gingen und dabei Zielobjekte einsammelten und/oder Hindernisse vermieden.

Wie erwartet, zeigte sich, dass unabhängig von der Objektkonfiguration und der aktuellen Aufgabe Blickverschiebungen in Richtung eines benachbarten

2

Objekts häufiger auftraten als Blickverschiebungen in die entgegengesetzte Richtung. Noch häufiger zeigte sich dieser Effekt, wenn das benachbarte Objekt aufgabenrelevant war. Letzteres erwies sich allerding nur für Situationen, in denen die Probanden beide Aufgaben (Zielobjekte sammeln und Hindernisse vermeiden) zeitgleich ausführen mussten, signifikant.

Diese Ergebnisse sind ein Hinweis darauf, dass periphere Informationen die Blickposition in realitätsnahen Aufgaben beeinflussen können. Zudem kann aufgrund des Effekts der Aufgabenrelevanz und damit verbundener Belohnung der hier gefundene Effekt als sinnvolle Blickstrategie interpretiert werden. Folglich sollte die exklusive Rolle des fovealen Sehens in Modellen zum menschlichen Blickverhalten überdacht werden.

1. Introduction

Think back to July 13th 2014, the final of the FIFA Soccer World Cup 2014 in the Maracanã stadium in Rio de Janeiro, Brazil. It is the 30th minute of play, the game is in full swing, and the scoreboard still shows a 0:0 between Germany and Argentina. Suddenly, a pass from the midfield reaches the Argentinian forward Ezequiel Lavezzi, who is all by himself on the right-hand side. Two Argentinian players, Gonzalo Higuain and Marcos Rojo, take their chance; they start sprinting towards the German penalty area trying to pull clear of the German defense. Lavezzi hoofs the ball forward. Benedikt Höwedes, a German defender, is not able to clear the ball, and Lavezzi crosses it towards the center. As it has often been the case in this tournament, it all comes down to the German goalkeeper Manuel Neuer to remedy the situation for the German team. But what is the best strategy for Neuer to clear the ball in this difficult situation?

The latter question is an example of what this study will be concerned with: Which strategy, in this particular case which strategy of gaze allocation, do people use in natural settings when confronted with multiple tasks and objects, which demand their attention?

Admittedly, being the German goalkeeper at the World Cup finals is not what the average person does in his everyday life, however, situations, in which we have to pay attention to several objects or tasks at once occur considerably often. Take, for instance, driving through bustling traffic in an unknown city: You have to be attentive not to crash into the car in front of you, but at the same time you are aware of the three kids playing ball on the sidewalk. Another example for such an everyday task is walking along the pedestrian precinct. You need to get where you are going while making sure not to run into other pedestrians or to step into a gum sticking on the ground.

Back to Manuel Neuer at the World Cup finals: What kinds of gaze strategies are conceivable in such a demanding and fast situation? Is only fixating and paying attention to the ball flying towards the center sensible? Of course, Neuer needs to know the ball's location to estimate its trajectory to be able to clear the ball. Nevertheless, should he not also be aware of his opponents' locations since it is possible that one of them receives the ball earlier than him? If Neuer is not aware of them, it might end terribly for the German team. Thus, there is some consent that visual attention is spread at least somehow. Hence, is it the "best" strategy to sequentially allocate gaze between the ball and the two opponents to know exactly where all three of them are located and what they are doing? This strategy sounds plausible, nevertheless it is also time consuming, since fixations lasts about 300msec on average. These fractions of a second can determine the difference between victory and defeat. Consequentially, the following questions arise: Is it likely that a less time consuming but also less accurate strategy is used in the sense of a tradeoff. For instance, is it beneficial to allocate one's gaze to an intermediate spot and as a result see all task relevant objects (i.e. the ball and the two opponents in this example) in the peripheral visual field at once?

This is what the present study will discuss. Does information of the peripheral visual field contribute to strategies of gaze allocation in everyday tasks? Which role does the task-relevance of objects in the periphery play? Moreover, should models of gaze allocation in naturalistic settings consider to integrate peripheral information in their predictions as well?

Before describing the methods and results of the present study, which examined the allocation of gaze and the influence of peripheral information in a virtual walking task, the next sections will give an overview about some essentials of foveal and peripheral vision (see section 1.1. Foveal and Peripheral Vision – Physiological and Functional Fundamentals). Then, the topic of visual attention will be addressed briefly (see section 1.2. A Brief Glance on the Subject of Visual Attention). Afterwards, this chapter will describe two confined exemplary concepts, one in the context of foveal vision, gaze allocation and natural settings (see section 1.3. The Allocation of Gaze in Natural Tasks) and one on how peripheral information can influence gaze (see section 1.4. An Effect of Peripheral Information on Gaze).

1.1. Foveal and Peripheral Vision – Physiological and Functional Fundamentals

The receptive surface within the human eye, the retina, consists of several neural layers. After light enters the eye through the pupil it has to pass the ganglion cell layer and a cell layer containing bipolar cells, amacrine cells, and horizontal cells, before it impinges on the photoreceptor cell layer (Kolb & Whishaw, 2001; Wandell, 1995). These photoreceptors, which contain light sensitive pigments, stop releasing neurotransmitters when incoming photons are absorbed. They can be classified into two separate kinds of receptors: rods and cones (Pinel, 2009). Rods are longer (Kolb & Whishaw, 2001), but smaller in diameter than cones (Wandell, 1995). While there about 100 million rods, only about 5 million cones are spread across the retina of each eye (Wandell, 1995). Rods have a higher sensitivity to light and can therefore be aroused by less light, for instance at night (scotopic vision), whereas cones work optimally under daylight conditions (photopic vision; Pinel, 2009). This lack in sensitivity of cones is counterbalanced with high visual acuity and perception of color, which in turn cannot be provided by rods (Pinel, 2009).

Rods and cones are not distributed evenly across the retina. The highest concentration of cones is found in the fovea, as the central region of the retina is termed (see below; Kolb & Whishaw, 2001). This peak decreases rapidly with increasing eccentricity from fovea (Pinel, 2009). Rods, on the other hand, are non-existing in the fovea, but numerous in non-foveal parts (Pinel, 2009).

Taken together, the fovea and the non-foveal parts of the retina serve different aspects in the process of visual perception. These differences are not only based on varying relative densities of rods and cones, but more importantly, are also due to differences in neural connections within the eye (Pinel, 2009). In general, photoreceptors are connected with bipolar cells, which in turn are linked

7

to retinal ganglion cells, that integrate the incoming information (Kolb & Whishaw, 1996). The differences in absolute sensitivity and visual acuity between foveal and peripheral vision are primarily due to differences in the convergence of receptors onto bipolar cells, and of bipolar cells onto ganglion cells. In the fovea the interconnection is exclusive: Considering a single ganglion cell, there are only a few cones each, which project onto it. This connectivity in the fovea scales down to the optimal limit, namely a one-to-one wiring between cones and ganglion cells (Gegenfurtner, 2006; Pinel, 2009). This non – or little – convergence (Wandell, 1995), results in high spatial resolution, since the brain gets information from the ganglion cells via the optic nerve and can deduce which photoreceptor in the fovea absorbed photons and in turn is able to compute the position of the light source to build up the field of view. That is why the fovea is the region of highest visual acuity (Kolb & Whishaw, 1996). In non-foveal or peripheral regions of the retina, the convergence of photoreceptors is higher: hundreds of rods can project on a single ganglion cell (Wandell, 1995). Consequently, if a ganglion cell is firing due to excitement of rods, the brain cannot infer which rod sent the initial signal. This in turn results in low visual acuity (Pinel, 2009).

To sum it up, due to the variations in the relative densities of different photoreceptor cells and their specific connectivity features, foveal vision provides high acuity while in peripheral vision a gradual decline in visual acuity with increasing distance from the fovea is recognizable.

Another reason for differences between foveal and non-foveal vision is the cortical representation. The primary visual cortex (V1 or Area Striata) is organized in a retinotopic fashion (Gegenfurtner, 2006), such as other parts of the visual stream. That means that neighboring locations on the retina are also located next to each other in V1. A special feature of this organization is that the fovea is overrepresented, that is, foveal and near foveal vision take up about 50 % of the whole primary visual cortex while the rest of the visual field needs to share the residual half of the cortical representation capacity (Gegenfurtner, 2006). This again shows the amount of importance granted to foveal vision. However, the significance of peripheral vision should not be understated. For instance, the perception of movement is developed more highly in peripheral than in foveal vision (Kolb & Whishaw, 2001).

To close this section on elementary differences, please note that the distinction made in the present study only distinguishes between foveal and non-foveal vision. The latter actually includes *parafoveal* and *peripheral* vision by definition (e.g. Wyszecki & Stiles, 2000). This further subdivision is not used here since the eccentricities of objects in the visual field were not quantified. Non-foveal vision is from here on referred to as *peripheral vision* for reasons of the reader's convenience.

The next section will give a short introduction on some aspects of visual attention.

1.2. A Brief Glance on the Subject of Visual Attention

In the context of the present study, it is important to know which role visual attention plays and how it can be spread across the visual field.

By definition, attention is the mechanism, by which processing capacity is assigned to a limited number of objects or tasks (Findlay, 2003). Attention is often described as a 'bottleneck', illustrating that this cognitive resource is limited at every given point in time. In visual attention, this bottleneck metaphor becomes even more apparent, since foveal vision – and by association the position of gaze – are tightly linked to the focus of visual attention (e.g. Hoffman & Subramaniam, 1995; Schneider & Deubel, 1995).

Several studies showed evidence for the coupling of saccadic eye movements and visual attention, for instance, Schneider and Deubel (1995), who examined the interaction of these two elements in a letter detection task. They randomly cued one position within one of two presented three-letter strings, to which the subject were instructed to make a saccade to. The middle letter of the cued three-letter string was changed to an 'E' or its mirrored version and the subjects had to detect which of the two were presented. The presentation of the target was held shortly, so that the saccade towards the cued position was initiated after the targets had disappeared. Their results revealed that the target discrimination was best when the position of the discrimination target was the same as the cued saccade position (Schneider & Deubel, 1995). The authors reasoned that the intention to make a saccade already shifts the attentional spotlight towards the saccadic target position and consequently facilitates perceptual tasks, such as letter detection.

This was also shown by the results of Hoffman and Subramaniam (1995). Moreover, they examined if subjects were able to make saccades to one particular target while attending another one. The subjects were instructed verbally which position they should pay attention to. However, this manipulation of attention allocation did not produce differences in their detection task. The only determining factor was if the saccadic target position and the position of the target presentation coincided or not. Again, the detection performance was best when the target was presented at the saccadic target position, although the target letter had already disappeared when subjects initiated the eye movement.

As an inversion of this argumentation, a large number of studies – especially the ones in which subjects are free to choose where to look – assume that a shift in a person's attention is reliably indicated by a shift of gaze. Based on the findings on coupling between attention and eye movements, this assumption is reasonable and a sensible simplification. Additionally, in every day conversations eye contact is taken as an indicator, if the dialog partner is paying attention or not. However, this definition is only one side of the coin since there is no one-to-one relation between gaze and attention.

To illustrate this idea, imagine the following situation: You are having dinner with a friend in a nice restaurant. She is talking about some trouble with her co-worker; you are keeping eye contact with her, nodding, and pretending to listen, although – to be honest – you are not very interested. Instead of listening to her complains, you are listening to the conversation on the neighbor table; the two men are talking about the latest news, which you find more interesting. This example shows that it is possible to fixate a certain object, such as a friend's face here, while paying auditory attention to something or someone else.

The same holds true for visual attention. Think back to the car-driving example at the beginning (see section 1. Introduction). You need to make sure not to crash into the car in front of you, so you will probably look at it. While fixating the car you are still able to pay attention to the children on the sidewalk, just in case one of them suddenly runs across the street. You do not necessarily have to look at the children to direct your attentional spotlight towards them.

The difference between these two daily situations and the findings on gaze-attention coupling described above is the crucial gaze variable: In experiments on visual attention, mainly eye *movements* are investigated; the examples in 'real-world' settings rather describe the intentional allocation of attention while keeping gaze *fixed*.

Empirical evidence, which shows that it is possible to decouple gaze and visual attention by holding a constant gaze position while accomplishing a given task, was shown in several experiments. Talking in terms of foveal and peripheral vision, this possibility of decoupling shows that information from the peripheral visual field can be used to accomplish purposeful tasks. This view was also held by Henderson, Pollatsek, and Rayner (1989) examining object identification performances. Subjects had to scan four objects in two different conditions and to decide afterwards, if a particular object was previously displayed or not. In one condition, all objects were shown at the same time on screen. In a second condition, only the currently fixated object was visible while the other three objects were masked. The mean fixation time spent on the single objects was longer when only one object was visible at a time. This suggests that peripheral information is used in the identification of objects when all of them are visible in the second condition. For further results on this topic, see Posner (1980).

The present study also takes up the question of exploitation of peripheral information. More specifically, not only the covert spreading of attention across the visual field is of interest, but also the influence on spatial gaze positions due to peripheral information. The assumption herein is that attention directed towards objects in the peripheral field can lead to a bias in gaze locations (see sections 1.5. The Paradigm and the Aim of the Study, and 1.6. Hypotheses and Implementation). A similar idea concerning microsaccades was investigated, for instance by Engbert and Kliegl (2003) as well as Hafed and Clark (2002).

As already mentioned above, the next section will be about one very particular approach in the framework of foveal vision. A model of scheduling gaze

11

allocation will be introduced, which focuses on predictions in natural tasks and for that reason makes usage of Virtual Reality set-ups.

1.3. The Allocation of Gaze in Natural Tasks

In recent years, a unique opportunity arose from advances in Computer Sciences, in the quality of portable eye tracking set-ups, and in the technology of conducting Virtual Reality (from now on referred to as VR). They have enabled researchers to model human behavior, to make these predictions tangible by virtual agents, and to investigate subjects' actual behavior in the same virtual environment while providing naturalistic tasks and experimental control at the same time (Rothkopf, Ballard, & Hayhoe, 2007). Furthermore, being able to study eye movements in more realistic tasks, whether in virtual or real world, makes it possible to draw further conclusions about the workings of human vision in everyday life. Section 1.3.1. *'Walter' – A Model of Scheduling Gaze Allocation* will describe one computational models attempting to predict human behavior, or more precisely, an attempt on how human gaze allocation can be scheduled. The subsequent section 1.3.2. *Findings on Human Behavior in Naturalistic Tasks using Virtual Reality* will then report results of experiments, which tested if the assumptions and predictions of the model are vindicated in human behavior during naturalistic tasks.

1.3.1. 'Walter' – A Model of Scheduling Gaze Allocation

One of the above-mentioned computational models that is taking advantage of virtual agents to test its predictions of where humans pay foveal attention to over extended time periods, was introduced by Sprague, Ballard, and Robinson (2007). This model of gaze scheduling is one of the first to take top-down processes, such as the agent's behavioral goals, into account and therefore give vision a purposeful role in naturalistic, temporally extended tasks that humans take part in every day (Hayhoe, Shrivastava, Mruczek, & Pelz, 2003; Land, Mennie, & Rusted, 1999). Hence, this model emphasizes several aspects, namely:

I)   Embodiment of Cognition
II)   Composition of Behavior
III)   A Hierarchical Structure
IV)   Reinforcement Learning
V)   A Special Role of Gaze.

This overview given here is strongly based on the descriptions and explanations given by Sprague et al. (2007). Since they refer to their own model as 'Walter', that is actually the artificial human, who is led through virtual environments by their algorithm, this eponym will also be used in the following to refer to this particular model of gaze allocation.

Each of the five characteristics will be explained in detail in the following sections (see sections 1.3.1.1. Embodiment of Cognition to 1.3.1.5. The Special Role of Gaze), starting with the principle of embodied and embedded cognition.

1.3.1.1. Embodiment of Cognition

One of the most fundamental assumptions of the Walter model is that vision takes place in a (human) being and cannot adequately be modeled separately from a (human) body that contains other systems as well (Ballard, Kit, Rothkopf, & Sullivan, 2013). This idea was already summarized by Andy Clark in 1999. According to his understanding of embodied cognition, cognitive processes could never be viewed as isolated: The brain, in which cognition takes places, is localized in the human body, which again is situated in a certain environment. Thereby, embodiment and environmental embeddedness provide both resources and constraints for human cognition and behavior (Clark, 1999; Firby, Kahn, Prokopowicz, & Swain, 1995). These can in turn be utilized actively and – at the most – successfully by humans to interact with their environment. Hence, knowing about the particular resources and constraints – and as a result the limited number of degrees of freedom – makes it considerably easier for both, the visual system itself to process information as well as researchers to model and predict human behavior (e.g. Ballard, Hayhoe, Pook, & Rao, 1997; Firby et al., 1995). For instance, in the context of building models for human saccades, it is not necessary to enable the model to predict thirty saccades per second, since it is known that the human oculomotor control system is usually capable of about three saccades per second (Goldstein, 2008).

The assumption of embodied cognition also yields a role of gaze different from the well-known four-step paradigm of Marr (1982). Marr suggested that the purpose of vision is to provide a retinal image of the surrounding world for creating primal and 2½-D sketches of it, to finally come to an *internal* 3-D model of the world for the human to work with. However, according to Clark (1999), vision plays a main role by being an "*active* retrieval [...] of useful information as it is needed from the constantly present real-world scene" (Clark, 1999, p. 346). Thus, the oculomotor system can be viewed as an 'intelligent' on-time provider of visual information to make the human able to interact with the external world (Clark, 1999, p. 346) and its demands over extended times.

Ballard et al. (1997) adapted this idea in their concept of deictic computations. They suggested that on a time scale of one third of a second, fixations (as well as hand movements like pointing) are used to directly connect *external* data about the environment to the current *internal* cognitive or behavioral goal. In this way, samples of information can be acquired sequentially just before they are needed for the next step of motor action to accomplish the current task.

It is important to note, that according to Walter, only the object feature (e.g. color, position, size, etc.) which is important for the current subtask is internally represented, that is, stored in visual working memory (Ballard, Hayhoe, & Pelz, 1995; see section 1.3.1.2. Composition of Behavior). One great advantage of these 'just-in-time representations' (Ballard et al., 1997, p. 739) is computational economy by not building up a complete model of the outer world. Such an extensive copy (Marr, 1982) might contain unnecessary information, which – in

14

terms of cognitive processing – is expensive to build up and to remember, especially if not needed. Thus, deictic coding allows the agent to use its environment as "cheap" 'external memory' (Ballard et al., 1995, p. 79).

After having explained the concepts of embodied cognition and deictic computations, the next principle addresses the segmentation of behavior.

1.3.1.2. Composition of Behavior

Walter is a compositionally built model of behavior (Sprague et al., 2007), which results in its central premise: Any behavior can be described by its constituent components and their related task plus the policy of their dynamic interaction (Ballard et al., 2013).

This principle follows the approach of Brooks (1986), who suggested a new control system for an autonomically working mobile robot. He claimed that complex behavior decomposed in simpler 'task achieving behaviors' is a robust way to represent the subdivision of behavior. Instead of subdividing behavior into functional modules of either perception, cognition *or* action (Marr, 1982; cited after Sprague et al., 2007), Brooks claimed that each behavior pattern consists of perception, cognition, *and* action. Hence, all three stages should be considered within this fundamental unit of describing complex behavior (cf. Figure 2B in Sprague et al., 2007). Those simple behaviors are thought to be sequentially tied together to achieve the agent's behavioral goals (Sprague et al., 2007).

The Walter model of Sprague et al. (2007) adopted Brooks' idea of task achieving tasks, labeling these sensory-motor behaviors 'microbehaviors'. They defined a microbehavior as "a complete sensory/motor routine that incorporates mechanisms for measuring the environment and acting on it to achieve specific goals" (p. 5).

As in Brooks' model (1986), a microbehavior is the minimum unit of behavior, meaning it is not possible to break it down into elements that are more basic. Further, the above-mentioned constraints caused by the premise of embodiment help limit these microbehaviors to a certain level of plainness (cf. Figure 3 in Sprague et al., 2007).

To illustrate the idea of microbehaviors, here are some examples used in previous experiments and in the present study: Imagine Walter is walking along a path, which has several objects on it. The microbehaviors for this situation could be to stay on the given path, to gather objects of interest, but also to avoid obstacles that might get in the way (see 2.3. Stimuli and Task). Further, assume that the microbehavior of avoiding obstacles is currently running while Walter is walking along the path. Walter would extract relevant information from the visual scene by directing his gaze towards an obstacle on his path. Relevant information in this case would be the size of the obstacle, his own position relative to the obstacle in three-dimensional space, the angle of approaching the obstacle or possible ways to navigate around it. Having information about the current state of the world, Walter can choose an action from a whole table of actions by indexing this table and sending the signal for the chosen action to his motor system for execution, for instance 'turn left for 10° to pass the obstacle on its left side'. This mapping process is assumed to be driven by reward maximization given the current estimate about the world. The concept of reward maximization for choosing and execution of actions is explained below in section 1.3.1.4. *Allocation of Foveal Attention in the Context of Reinforcement Learning.*

Throughout this process of updating the current state, choosing, and executing behavior, the currently active set of microbehaviors must be updated appropriately. The model assumes that more than a single, but only a limited number of microbehaviors can be active at once (Ballard et al., 2013). In this context, the authors refer to the limited number of processed features in visual working memory (Luck & Vogel, 1997). A study, which showed that subjects use very limited memory capacity in accomplishing tasks when free to choose their own strategy, was conducted by Ballard et al. in 1995. In a virtual block pattern copy task, subjects were presented a model of several blocks in four different colors (model area) and were asked to rebuild it as quickly and accurately as possible. No further instruction was given. In the resource area, a pool of blocks of each color was held available for the subjects to work with, while a workspace area was provided as space for the rebuilding. Four patterns of fixation strategies were observed frequently across subjects, which were interpreted in terms of the extent of using visual working memory capacity. For instance, one strategy was thought to indicate that there is no memorization of the block's color or position since both are rechecked just before the information was needed in the course of the task Intriguingly, the results revealed that the relative frequencies of total strategy usage were highest for the 'no memorization' strategy (Ballard et al., 1995). This indicates that subjects try to minimize their workload in visual working memory by extracting important information via multiple fixations. These results go hand in hand with the idea of fixations used as deictic codes in natural tasks (Ballard et al., 1997), as described in section 1.3.1.1. *Embodiment of Cognition*. They suggested that crucial data about the environment is gathered by fixating task-relevant properties of the image instantaneously before performing an action.

To further substantiate their interpretation of compensating expensive memory representations Ballard et al. (1995) conducted an adjoining study varying the cost of making fixations by forcing subjects to increase saccades or respectively to make even larger head movements. This was implemented by varying the distance between the model and the workspace area. In conditions in which the deictic coding was more expensive due to distance, subjects tended to use fixation patterns based on memory more often than before. This undermines the idea of economical compromises between making fixations and visual working memory. Still, the usage of the latter seems to be limited and since Sprague et al. (2007) assume that the number of active microbehaviors is related to the capacity of visual working memory, it is thought to be limited as well. However, the exact number is arguable.

Returning to the idea of microbehaviors, it is important to mention that although a set of several microbehaviors can be *active* at the same time (e.g. stay on path, collect target objects, and avoid obstacles), only one single micro-behavior can be updated by the current input and as a consequence carried out at any given point in time. The currently not updated microbehaviors maintain an estimate based on previous information. Thus, the independent tasks are updated in a serial manner by allocating gaze to the task relevant locations (Sullivan, Johnson, Rothkopf, Ballard, & Hayhoe, 2012).

To control these updating processes, a hierarchical architecture was built into the Walter model, which will be described next.

17

1.3.1.3. Hierarchical Control Structure

Like former models of behavior (e.g. Brooks, 1986; Firby et al., 1995), the model of Sprague et al. (2007) is hierarchically designed and akin to the conceptualization of Firby et al. (1995).

In their 'Animate Agent Architecture', Firby et al. (1995) emphasized the idea of efficiency in a variety of tasks by lowering the complexity of visual problems and the reusability of basic modules. They claimed that the simplification of visual problems is achieved by utilization of as many constraints as possible that naturally occur from the environment and the agent's task. Providing this information of constraints on a high level, their model is able to dynamically adapt to changing environments and tasks by combining its basic elements in an environment- and task-*specific* way. The purpose of visual routines in this context is to provide required task-specific visual information. Action routines are simply the implementation of behaviors deemed appropriate in the particular situation when one considers the current constraints. To ensure the success of the model while performing actions in real-time, it also contains a control system, which updates free parameters to current, unexpected, changes in the environment. The usage of currently perceived information is necessary to adapt the execution of actions and consequently to produce more reliable behavior in real-time. That also means that this control system can terminate a currently running skill if it does not meet the present challenges, and start another, more appropriate skill for the situation.

Revisiting the Walter model by Sprague et al. (2007), their model also focuses on the appropriate adaptability to altering demands of the environment and the agent's task by running the analogous microbehavior in real-time (Sprague et al., 2007). Thus, information about the agent's current situation provided by the vision system needs to be translated into goal-achieving motor commands in an on-line fashion. Therefore, they describe a hierarchy of allocating resources as follows.

The Walter model is structured hierarchically into three levels: (a) a *behavior level,* (b) an *arbitration level,* and (c) a *context level.* This structure inevitably results in new roles for vision in the scheduling and running of goal-specific subtasks (see below).

The model's level of individual behavior is responsible for running active microbehaviors (see section 1.3.1.2. Composition of Behavior), each of which needs and gets information derived from perceptional mechanisms. The role of gaze allocation at this stage is to provide this necessary state information in real time. Since this information about the environment is changing constantly due to the agent's action, the visual computation needs to be done rapidly. This is possible, because goal-specific computations are considerably simpler and therefore less time-consuming than those computations, which do not consider the current task (Sprague et al., 2007).

The second level is the arbitration level. As explained above, several microbehaviors can be active at the same time, forming a *set* of active microbehaviors. Thus, since they are embodied in the same agent, they have to share limited resources. The role of arbitration at this stage is to solve the conflicting demands between them. The body's limited resources need to be allocated to certain microbehaviors. These are recommended by the behavior level incorporating the current state of the agent on the one hand, and critical goals of the agent in the current context (see context level below) on the other hand.

The role of vision on the arbitration level is to allocate gaze to a spatial position on which the least loss of reward (see section 1.3.1.4. Allocation of Foveal Attention in the Context of Reinforcement Learning) is expected. It is assumed that this happens rather sequentially for different microbehaviors than to allow the possibility of a "shared fovea" between the microbehaviors of the currently active set. That means that each fixation is assumed to conduce only the one running microbehavior, respectively the analogous sub-task, at each point in time. It is necessary to keep this assumption in mind, since this constitutes an oversimplification, which is questioned in the present study (see section 1.5. The Paradigm and the Aim of the Study).

The hierarchy's most abstract level is the context level. As its name implies, at this stage, the processing and decisions of the two lower levels are judged at their adequacy in the greater context. In particular, every 300 milliseconds the presently active set of microbehaviors is evaluated, if it meets the demands of the current goals of the agent and the external circumstances.

Now, that the allocation of gaze was described in the greater context of the model's hierarchy, it is sensible to explain which "driving forces" underlie the sequential redirecting of foveal attention.

1.3.1.4. Allocation of Foveal Attention in the Context of Reinforcement Learning

The questions of how Walter chooses the next action from the available possibilities and how the next position of gaze allocation is selected can be answered in connection with a reward maximization framework. Therefore, the authors used a standard *Q-learning* algorithm as mathematical feedback tool in the simulation of behavior (Sullivan et al., 2012). For further details on the mathematical approach and the specific computations, see Ballard et al. (2013), Rothkopf and Ballard (2013), and Sprague et al. (2007).

The mapping from current states to appropriate actions is accomplished by choosing the action for which the highest reward is expected. For eye movements – as a special case of human behavior since they provide infor-mation rather than change the circumstances in a desirable way – there cannot be an immediate reinforcement (except for some social settings [Sullivan et al., 2012]), which would be necessary for learning according to the theory of reinforcement learning (Skinner, 1938). Although immediate reward for gaze behavior is unlikely in natural situations, research has shown that the oculomotor control system is set for value-based modulations. For instance, Schütz, Trommershäuser, and Gegenfurtner (2012) investigated the impact of salience and value in a saccade task. They showed subjects stimuli consisting of three blended parts of different luminance. These parts were ascribed different values in three conditions: in the first condition, no values were assigned; in the second condition, one part was defined as the reward area (resulting in monetary recompense after the experiment when making saccades to it); in the third condition, the reward area was defined as well as a penalty area (resulting in a subtraction of monetary recompense). Their results revealed that saccadic landing positions depended on both salience and value. In the first condition in which the values of the stimuli parts were not defined, salience was the determining factor of saccadic landing positions. In the remaining two conditions, it was a question of saccadic latency which of these factors was taken more into account in the programming of saccades. The results suggested that in cases of quick saccades, salience outweighed value, whereas value was given more weight when subjects took longer time for the programming of saccades as indicate by longer latencies. Comparable results were obtained by Stritzke, Trommershäuser, and Gegenfurtner (2009).

Nevertheless, the authors of the model claim, that in real-life situations values, which are ascribed to gaze allocation, are associated with other actions that might be rewarded after executing. These actions are again the ones chosen and executed within the microbehavior unit (Ballard et al., 2013).

Another relevant factor that the model considers is uncertainty (Sullivan et al., 2012; Tong & Hayhoe, 2014). Since the information provided by the human senses, respectively vision in this case, is not always perfect, a certain degree of uncertainty about the current state remains (Sullivan et al., 2012). This non-perfect estimate of the current state might cause costs by executing actions, which do not result in a maximum reward. This costs needs to be avoided by making "correct" fixations. In terms of reward learning, the amount of positive loaded reward is reduced and therefore the frequency of "incorrect" fixations should be decreased. Thus, gaze is allocated to positions that will minimize the negative costs of uncertainty and consequently maximize the expected reward.

In the context of experimentally investigating implicit reward, it is assumed that it can be reliably varied by the task and its priority accomplished by instructions (Sullivan et al., 2012). That means that when subjects are told to carry out a certain task, the subject's reward, which motivates the particular actions, is simply the accomplishment of the task itself.

The last characteristic of the Walter model, which is the most important principle in the context of the present study, will address why foveal vision is assigned a very special role.

1.3.1.5. The Special Role Of Gaze

Resulting from the considerations described above, vision and especially foveal vision is accredited an exceptional role in human behavior. From evolutionary, psychological, and neuroscientific research it is known that humans are predominantly "visual creatures". That is, humans rely heavily on visual information, even if additional information is provided by other perceptual systems, such as haptic or auditory input (Ernst & Bülthoff, 2004).

However, the role of vision going along with the assumptions of the Walter model is special since up to its publication previous models had focused on explaining human visuomotor behavior, like gaze allocation, in the context of bottom-up processing. Bottom-up models like those of salience (e.g. Itti & Koch, 2000) consider image features such as color or contrast, to be the main aspects in driving gaze by a precedent shift of visual attention (see section 1.2. A Brief Glance on the Subject of Visual Attention). In contrast, several recent studies have shown that those kind of salience models do not make reliable predictions of human gaze allocation in a variety of tasks, especially in naturalistic tasks (Rothkopf et al., 2007; Sprague et al., 2007; Tong & Hayhoe, 2014).

The Walter model takes into account effects of the agent's cognitive goal in the current task, which is profoundly associated with a maximization of implicit reward (see section 1.3.1.4. Allocation of Foveal Attention in the Context of Reinforcement Learning). Therefore, gaze allocation is regarded as purposeful within mainly top-down driven processes (Sprague et al., 2007).

Evidence for the usage of top-down processes in the allocation of gaze was given, among others, by Neider and Zelinsky (2006). They let subjects search for jeeps, helicopters, blimps, or fictional objects in a 3D desert scene. Subjects were not enabled to walk through the virtual scene. Their results show that subjects relied on pre-existing knowledge and scene context during the search, since they were searching for blimps in the sky and jeeps on the ground, which is reasonable due to their real-life expected occurrence. Fictional objects and helicopters were presented either in the sky or on the ground, each in 50% of trials. The difference between these two is that prior knowledge is only available for the helicopter; and this seemed to make the difference. Since there can be no knowledge based expectation for the occurrence of the fictional object, the results showed no meaningful search preference for sky or ground. At the same time, when searching for a helicopter there was a preference to look towards the sky region of the visible scene, which suggests that top-down processes, such as knowledge, influence gaze behavior.

In this top-down processing framework, the authors of Walter make a clear distinction between foveal and peripheral vision: The Walter model explicitly assumes that visual information is gathered from only one point at a time, which is the fixated part of the visual scene. Further, this information is used only for the currently running microbehavior, or subtask. Several findings support this idea (e.g. Ballard et al., 1995; Shinoda, Hayhoe, & Shrivastava, 2001; Rothkopf et al., 2007; Sullivan et al., 2012; see section 1.3.2. Findings on Human Behavior in Naturalistic Tasks using Virtual Reality). Still, this assumption is undoubtedly a simplification in the context of visual attention (see section 1.2. A Brief Glance on the Subject of Visual Attention).

To exaggerate this premise in terms of visual attention, the model would suggest that the focus of attention is not only indicated by the position of gaze, but that the foveated region is the *only* spot in the visual field attention can be paid to at any given point in time. Taken for granted and as already pointed out in section 1.2. *A Brief Glance on the Subject of Visual Attention*, the center of gaze is tightly linked to the center of attention in a variety of contexts (Hoffman & Subramaniam, 1995; Schneider & Deubel, 1995) and is therefore an useful indicator of current cognitive processes. Nevertheless, it is possible to spread attention peripheral parts of the visual filed and to use visual information gathered from these non-foveal parts (Henderson et al., 1989; Posner, 1980).

This idea was already touched in the Manuel Neuer example (see section 1. Introduction). Although we might not directly fixate on a particular object in the visual scene, it is possible to direct our attention towards this object in the peripheral visual field. In the example at the outset, this means that the goalkeeper has to pay attention to the two approaching opponents while looking at the ball or respectively at some point of its estimated trajectory (for findings on trajectory estimates in a racket ball task, see Diaz, Cooper, Rothkopf, & Hayhoe, 2013).

The premise of the exclusive role of foveal vision has been made for two reasons: First, there is no small amount of findings suggesting that fixations, and hence foveal vision, play a very special role in natural tasks. For instance, Ballard et al. (1995) found in an extended version of their block copying experiment, that if subjects were asked to hold their gaze fixed on a predefined spot between the model, the resource, and the workspace area, they could accomplish the copy task, but vastly slower than when being allowed to make saccades as they like to.

Secondly, since there are fewer parameters to estimate, predictions are simplified. Additionally, the findings on both virtual agent simulations as well as behavioral experiments testing the model's assumptions show that the model's predictions for gaze allocation are indeed quite veridical (see section 1.3.2. Findings on Human Behavior in Naturalistic Tasks using Virtual Reality). Thus, although the model does not consider parameters like attention to the peripheral visual field, it provides a broad framework for the workings of the visual system in everyday life.

It is important to mention that in the Walter model, this 'non-compromise' idea (see section 1.3.1.3. Hierarchical Control Structure) is only assumed for gaze allocation, but not for the executed actions: fixations can only update one microbehavior at a time, which happens every 300msec. The particular microbehavior gets new visual information while the other active, but not running microbehaviors have to rely on their possibly obsolete estimates. However, since actions are executed over extended times they can be a compromise between different active microbehaviors.

Following the description of the fundamentals and the determinants of the Walter model by Sprague et al. (2007) and before returning to the idea of non-compromising gaze and questioning the appropriateness of this premise, the next section will present some empirical findings of studies examining predictions and assumptions of the Walter model regarding reward learning and gaze's special role in natural behavior.

1.3.2. Findings on Human Behavior in Naturalistic Tasks using Virtual Reality

Turning now to the question of evidence or at least endorsement for Walter's assumptions, Sprague et al. (2007) examined if humans show task-related gaze patterns in a virtual navigation task as their model predicted. Six subjects had to walk along a virtual sidewalk, which they were told to stay on throughout the experiment. Distributed on this sidewalk were blue and purple blocks. The blue ones were obstacles that the subject should avoid, that is, trying not to walk through these blocks. The purple colored blocks were referred to as 'litter', which the subjects were asked to collect by walking through them. To make a more specific reference to the theoretical background of the model described above, these three task-related behaviors, namely 'stay on path', 'avoid blue obstacles', and 'collect purple litter', were thought to be the three microbehaviors (active set) competing for the deployment of gaze. Indeed, nearly all fixations made by subjects could be interpreted as conducing one of the tasks. Gaze was directed to the path or to one of the objects, rather than to other visual parts of the virtual environment. In addition, the authors examined if this pattern of gaze fixations can be explained by salience effects. They compared their data to prediction by the salience model of Itti and Koch (2000), which could not explain the data pattern, even with a fairly progressive comparison criterion. Sprague et al. (2007) interpreted these results as evidence for task-driven visual routines. However, it is important to mention that these results are no verification of the model (due to its complexity), but at least the human data showed the expected pattern (Sprague et al., 2007). Gaze patterns, which could be interpreted in terms of serving specific task-relevant purposes in natural tasks, have also been reported for making a peanut butter jelly sandwich (Land et al., 1999) and for brewing tea (Hayhoe et al., 2003).

Another study by Rothkopf et al. (2007), using the same sidewalk paradigm with blue and purple blocks and the collect litter and avoid obstacles tasks, further examined the role of different task combinations, different task priorities, salient but non task-relevant objects, and different arrangements of objects on gaze allocation. The subjects were instructed at the beginning of each trial, if they had to collect the litter, avoid the obstacles, or do both tasks simultaneously.

25

The resulting differences in the proportional fixation time between tasks showed that the task-relevance influenced gaze, in such a way that the proportional fixation time on a certain kind of object was higher, when the object was relevant in the current task. In the collect litter and the "both at once" condition, proportions of fixation time spent on litter objects were obviously the highest, with a slightly higher result (more than half of all fixations) in the former. In the avoid obstacles task, the proportional fixation time on litter objects dropped to the level of those on obstacle and the sidewalk. The two latter were fixated more often in the avoid obstacles condition than in the other conditions, yet, even in this condition the proportional time spent on litter was higher than the proportional time of fixations on obstacles. The relative time spent on objects in the background (e.g. buildings) was minor across all tasks. Overall, the fixation times differed significantly between the collect litter and the avoid obstacles task, but the comparisons with the "both at once" task did not.

In a further condition, in which the subjects also had to accomplish both tasks at the same time, additional highly salient objects (e.g. very colorful or moving objects) were presented in the virtual environment. Proportional time of fixations spent on these kind of objects was very small averaged across the trial. Only when not currently executing one of the tasks, which is at the beginning or the end of the walkway, relative fixation time spent on salient objects increased. Predictions of a salience-based model were computed to see if the data pattern can be explained by this kind of bottom-up processes. Again, the comparison did not yield persuasive results (Rothkopf et al., 2007), showing that the data of gaze patterns could not be explained by mere salience.

In the same series of experiments, Rothkopf et al. (2007) conducted an additional condition, in which all target and obstacle blocks were arranged *narrower* along the path. Most intriguingly in the context of the current study, the proportion of fixations made to the sidewalk dropped from 18% in the previous condition, in which the objects were arranged in a wider manner along the path, to only 4% in the narrower condition. Rothkopf et al. (2007) argued that fixations on targets and obstacles can in turn be interpreted as doing "double duty" by helping the subject to navigate along the path. They object to the interpretation of using peripheral vision for navigation, since the proportion of fixations should not be affected if this was the case.

Another interesting result reported by Rothkopf et al. (2007) is the difference in gaze distribution depending on the type of object and the related task. In the case of fixating litter objects in the collect litter task, subjects tended to look at the object center whereas when fixating obstacles in the avoidance task, gaze seemed to be distributed more densely around the object edge and more often on the bottom half (cf. Figure 6 in Rothkopf et al., 2007).

With regard to the idea of just-in-time, representations (Ballard et al., 1997) and thereby arising on-demand processing of visual information (see section 1.3.1.1. Embodiment of Cognition), Triesch, Hayhoe, Ballard, and Sullivan (2003) investigated if subjects detected changes in stimulus features as a function of their relevance to the current task. A virtual object-sorting task was conducted, in which the subjects had to pick up small blocks and put them down onto one of two conveyer belts depending on the current experimental condition. The three conditions used here differed in the task relevance of the block size: In one condition the size of the blocks did not matter at all; in the second condition, size only matters during the pick-up part of the task; and in the third condition, size mattered during picking up and while putting it down on the conveyer belt. The vertical size of the virtual blocks was changed during subjects' saccades between the picking up and putting down stage, so that subjects could only recognize the change when looking at the block again after it had changed. Interestingly, this change in size was recognized by subjects more often when the size of the block mattered for the specific task *after* it had changed, that is in the third condition, when size was relevant for the choice of the conveyer belt. These differences could not be explained by differing gaze patterns between the three conditions. Hence, the authors concluded that these differences might arise from differences in central processing modulated by task relevance of object features.

Differences due to task relevance were also found by Shinoda et al. (2001). In a virtual driving task subjects had to either follow a lead car or to follow the lead car while keeping track of the general traffic rules. Contrary to the study by Triesch et al. (2003), the participants knew which task was currently relevant.

This can explain why in the study of Shinoda et al. (2001) differences in gaze patterns were found between conditions. Here, scheduling of gaze allocation was affected by the current task, or respectively the cognitive goal of the subject. The results revealed that when subjects had to observe the general traffic rules, they made more fixations towards the side of the road, where traffic signs are visible in real life and towards intersections that they were approaching.

A similar experiment, which made usage of a driving simulator, was conducted by Sullivan et al. in 2012. They investigated the influence of reward and uncertainty on gaze predicted by the Walter model in a virtually simulated driving task. Subjects were instructed to follow a lead car while keeping the velocity of their car around a given speed limit. The priorities of these two tasks were manipulated by verbal instructions at the beginning of each trial, prioritizing one over the other. As explained above, implicit reward was thought to be manipulated by instruction and the desire of the subject to accomplish the given task. The variation of uncertainty was ensured by adding unpredictable noise to the car's gas pedal and the virtually shown speedometer in one half of the trials. The proportion of fixations on the speedometer and the lead car was greatly influenced by task priority and uncertainty: The proportional fixations on each of the two objects were higher when the object was relevant in the prioritized task (i.e. lead car in the following task, speedometer in the constant speed task). Additionally, uncertainty provided by noise was countered by proportional increase in fixations on the speedometer, but only if the task was to keep up to the constant speed limit, not while prioritizing the lead car task. Thus, only when the speed parameter was relevant to accomplish the task, gaze was deployed more often to fixations on the speedometer. Especially when noise made the estimates less reliable, relatively more fixations needed to be made to the speedometer to reduce the uncertainty in the current estimates of state (Sullivan et al., 2012).

The next paragraphs will describe the experiment, which the current study is directly associated with. This experiment was conducted by Tong and Hayhoe in 2014. Subjects walked along a winding path through a virtual room with blue spheres and brown obstacles arranged along the path. Eye movement data and body movement data were assessed in four different tasks: The subjects had to follow the path only, to collect blue target spheres, to avoid brown obstacle cubes or to collect the targets while avoiding the obstacles. In the three latter conditions, the subjects were instructed to stay close to the path, indicated by a light grey line on the floor. Unlike the current study, Tong and Hayhoe (2014) additionally manipulated the uncertainty about the virtual objects by letting them be stationary at one position (low uncertainty) or enabling them to move around (high uncertainty). Consequently, four different conditions were examined: stationary targets and stationary obstacles (low uncertainty for both object types); stationary targets and moving obstacles (low uncertainty for targets, high uncertainty for obstacles); moving targets and stationary obstacles (high uncertainty for targets, low uncertainty for obstacles); or moving targets and moving obstacles (low uncertainty for both object types).

For the number of contacted objects the following data pattern was revealed. As expected, in the collect targets task more targets than obstacles (which were declared as neutral or task irrelevant in this case) were contacted, while in the avoid obstacles task fewer obstacles than targets (task irrelevant) were made contact to. When subjects had to accomplish both tasks at the same time, that is, both object types are relevant to their corresponding task, more targets than obstacles were contacted. In addition, the number of collected targets was smaller than in the task, in which participants only had to keep track of collecting targets, as was the number of contacted obstacles, which were task relevant in the first but not in the latter. The results for the avoided obstacles in the "do both at once" task depicted no significant differences from the avoid obstacle condition: about the same small number of obstacles was contacted in the two tasks. In sum and in terms of relevance, more targets were made contact to when they were relevant than if they were not. The expected reversed data pattern was obtained for obstacles, that is less obstacles were contacted when they relevant to the current task than when they were not.

Besides the number of contacted objects, Tong and Hayhoe (2014) also examined the patterns of proportional fixations on the different kinds of objects in the different tasks and uncertainty conditions. The proportion of fixations on the path was the highest in the follow path task. Fixations on targets and on obstacles were made significantly more often when they were relevant to the current task than when they were not. The uncertainty factor did not influence the proportion of fixations on targets; there was no difference between stationary and moving targets, although moving objects are viewed as more salient. However, uncertainty did play a role in the proportional fixations on obstacles: When obstacles were task relevant, relatively more fixations were made on them when they were moving than when they had been stationary. No such difference between high and low uncertainty conditions were found, when obstacles were irrelevant for the task.

In addition, Tong and Hayhoe (2014) found that high numbers of collected targets were positively correlated with the proportional number of target fixations, while contacts with obstacles were negatively correlated with obstacle fixations, suggesting a more adequate performance in both tasks due to fixations.

All the results presented in this section show that the gaze allocation model by Sprague et al. (2007) makes reasonable assumptions and solid predictions for actual human behavior and therefore provides a suitable framework for further investigation of human vision in natural tasks. Nevertheless, as mentioned before, the constraint of only considering foveal and ignoring peripheral information will be questioned in the following. Therefore, the next chapter will introduce a well-known example of peripheral information influencing the location, to which people direct their gaze, namely the *visual center of gravity effect*.

1.4. An Effect of Peripheral Information on Gaze

The assumption that each of Walter's fixations only serves one certain task at a time (see section 1.3.1.5. The Special Role of Gaze) was scrutinized by the author while reviewing video data from a previous VR experiment conducted by *The Center of Perceptual Systems* at *The University of Texas at Austin*. The experiment examined the effect of reward and uncertainty on visuomotor behavior while walking through a virtual laboratory (similar to the experiment of Tong and Hayhoe (2014). Subjects seemed to show a tendency to make fixations to the wall behind some visible objects – formerly interpreted as stabilization fixations. However, in the context of the Walter model described above, these gaze locations do not serve a particularly important task since they do not provide useful state information. Taking into account that there were also fixations on objects with a tendency towards the object edge where other objects were visible in the periphery, the former can be seen as fixations on intermediate spot between several objects. Thus, the concept pursued here is that information of the peripheral visual field influences gaze position (see section 1.5. The Paradigm and the Aim of the Study for details). Before outlining the paradigm based on this idea, an overview of findings on this kind of fixation patterns will be given, since they have already been described in the context of object location research as so-called *center of gravity* or *center of mass* effects (e.g. Coren & Hoenig, 1972; Findlay, 1982; Hirsch & Mjolsness, 1992).

1.4.1. The Visual Center of Gravity – Defining the Concept

From a merely physical vantage point, the terms 'center of gravity' and 'center of mass' can be used synonymously when gravity can be assumed to be consistent (Nave, 2012). This is a reasonable assumption in the context of experiments taking place in a laboratory on earth. The center of gravity or center of mass (in the following taken together and shortened to COG) is an "imaginary point in a body of matter where [...] the total weight of the body may be thought to be concentrated" (Encyclopaedia Britannica, 2014). This body of matter can be a single object or a system of several objects, for which the COG is the center of the mass distribution averaging the masses weighted by their spatial distance (Nave, 2012).

In the context of looking at objects and preceding planning and execution of saccades, a number of approaches to qualify a visual COG has been suggested by object location research in the past (Guez, Marchal, Le Gargasson, Grall, & O'Regan, 1994; Hess & Holliday, 1992; Hirsch & Mjolsness, 1992; McGowan, Kowler, Sharma, & Chubb, 1998; Whitaker, McGraw, Pacey, & Barrett, 1996). In general, studies that investigated the characteristics of the visual COG effect's

31

expression seemed to avoid a strict definition of it. They rather described it loosely: Gaze allocation is influenced in some way by information of the currently visible scene, which results in saccadic landing errors, that is, saccades do not land on a target itself, but rather on a location between several targets or respectively between targets and distractors.

Nevertheless, a great diversity of approaches has been suggested trying to explain which visual feature of the stimuli configuration the visual COG is based on, for instance the maximum of the stimuli's contrast distribution (Hess & Holliday, 1992), or the average of the luminance distribution (Hirsch & Mjolsness, 1992).

Before reviewing some of the best-known results on the visual COG effect, its characteristics, and variations, some of these approaches will be introduced for better understanding in the following section (adapted from the overview given by Vishwanath & Kowler, 2003).

1.4.2. Approaches to a Visual Center of Gravity

One fairly simple and therefore attractive approach, since it assumes a pooling mechanism on an early visual stage, that is the retina (Vishwanath & Kowler, 2003), is defining the visual COG as the weighted mean of the luminance distribution of the present target configuration. For instance, Hirsch and Mjolsness (1992) tested three different models (Weber's law, window-of-attention and visual COG) to fit subjects' data in a random dot displacement discrimination task. Varying several parameters of the target configuration, their results showed that the dependent variable, the fractional JND (= *just noticeable difference*) for a given number of displaced dots, could be predicted best by the global spatial parameter provided by their visual COG model in contrast to the local spatial parameters of the other two models. They proposed two stages for the discrimination of moving direction: First, the computation of the global COG of the luminance distribution of the displayed dot configuration and second, a decision level (Hirsch & Mjolsness, 1992). Thus, a comparison between the visual COGs before and after dots are displaced is most helpful for reliable discrimination in this task.

Further endorsement for the approach of computing the COG based on luminance was given by findings of Whitaker et al. (1996). In a three-element Vernier alignment task, they found that for luminance-defined Gaussian blobs the COG of luminance is a good predictor for perceptual localization. Nevertheless, they also found that for higher-order stimuli, for instance Gabor and texture patches – which are not determined by sheer luminance, but by contrast – the COG of luminance is not a reliable predictor of human performance. Whitaker et al. (1996) suggested the usage of a 'centroid of the contrast envelope' for computation of perceived location instead, that is analogously the average of the contrast distribution of the presented target configuration.

This usage of the contrast distribution for the computation of the visual COG was upheld by the results of Guez et al. (1994). They conducted a study, in which the subjects had to count the corners of 12 differently shaped polygons with corners being shown or removed. By this task, the authors made sure that subjects made saccades to every corner of the presented polygon. What they found is that fixations towards the corners were influenced by the size of the angle, with average saccades closer to the corner for smaller angles than for larger angles. Additionally, this effect was influenced by corners being present or removed, showing mean landing positions closer to the corner for closed angles.

Three different COG models were fitted to the eye movement data and contrasted to differentiate, which of them could best predict the results found in this study. Those three models were the COG of luminance, the COG of contrast (as described above), and a COG of high curvature, which seems reasonable for the geometric stimuli that they used. Again, the best data fit was provided by the COG of contrast distribution (Guez et al., 1994).

Other research groups questioned the usage of sheer luminance or contrast distribution for perceived location, since these approaches might not be reliable in natural scenes. Like Hirsch and Mjolsness (1992), McGowan et al. (1998) presented random dot targets at three different eccentricities either left or right of a fixation cross. The subjects were asked to look at the target 'as a whole', whose midpoint laid on the same x-axis as the fixation cross. Further, subjects had to try to avoid corrective saccades and to take some time to initiate the change of gaze. The latter was thought to increase precision of the saccadic landing position. Again, saccadic landing positions were biased towards the horizontal COG of the random dot configuration, here defined as the mean of the horizontal coordinates of each dot in the presented pattern. In addition, McGowan et al. (1998) asked if it is possible to enhance the prediction of saccadic landing position by testing different models using a weighted mean instead of only using the unweighted mean as described above. Four different functions of spatial weights were suggested. First, a model of eccentricity dependence, assigning less weight to each point with increasing eccentricity. Second, a model of center accentuation, assigning the mean of a Gaussian function to the horizontal midpoint of the pattern. Third, a model of center attenuation, assigning an inverse Gaussian function to the horizontal midpoint of the pattern. And last, a model of neighbor proximity, assigning more weight to dots that did not have direct neighbors than to those dots that did. The results showed that only the weighted visual COG model described last led to a significant enhancement of predictions compared to the unweighted mean. Thus, it seems that single points in a random dot pattern are taken more into account in the planning of saccades (and therefore more weighted in the computation of the visual COG), when they were not surrounded by immediate neighboring dots (McGowan et al., 1998). They interpreted these results as evidence for the overall shape of the dot configuration being the crucial basis for the computation of the visual COG (McGowan et al., 1998, cited after Vishwanath & Kowler, 2003).

Still, the feature on which the visual COG effect is grounded remains arguable. Nevertheless, a variety of experiments was conducted to examine which factors can influence the COG. Some examples will be given hereafter.

1.4.3. Findings on the Visual Center of Gravity Effect

Two of the first researchers to describe center of gravity effects in the context of human vision were Coren and Hoenig in 1972. The results of their experiments
34

showed that for single-point stimuli the position of the first voluntary saccade towards a target was biased towards other non-target points in the periphery. Subjects had to make saccades from a fixation point to a target point shifted 10° on the horizontal axis. Coren and Hoenig varied the number and distance of up to three non-target points either between fixation point and target or on the outer side of the target.

In their first experiment, the non-target stimuli on either side of the target biased the landing position of the initial saccade towards themselves: Longer saccades were made in trials with outer non-target stimuli; shorter saccades were made in trials with inner non-target stimuli. Further, this bias was stronger the greater the number of non-target stimuli displayed.

In a second experiment, Coren and Hoenig (1972) tested if this saccade bias was due to the simple presence of the non-targets or to the consideration of a visual COG effect. For that purpose, they used the set-up explained above, with only one non-target stimulus and varied its distance to the target between trials. They demonstrated that with increasing non-target to target distance, the bias of the initial saccade towards the target increased too. Additionally, this effect was only applicable up to 4-6° non-target to target distance, shown by a massive drop of gaze bias for non-targets at a greater angle than this critical value. Besides that, if the non-target stimulus was shown between the fixation point and the target, the bias of the target-directed saccade was stronger than if the non-target stimulus was shown on the outer side of the target. They suggested that this might be due to the more accurate visibility of objects near the fovea.

Further examination of this effect was conducted by Findlay (1982), who coined the term *global effect* in this context. He defined this term as "[...] the idea that the information being used in the calculation of saccade amplitude is obtained by integrating information over a large spatial 'window'" (p. 1034). He further claimed that the global effect – although it can be affected by certain characteristics of the visual scene – is thought to be omnipresent. That is, foveal and non-foveal information is integrated in the process of saccade planning, but the latter might not become traceable for some systematically varied target configurations.

In his experiments, he was able to replicate the results of Coren and Hoenig (1972) to the effect that saccades towards two-target configurations landed on positions between them. In one of the experiments Findlay conducted in 1982, the subjects were asked to make saccades to a target configuration, consisting of either one or two single points, appearing sequentially at one of several unpredictable positions on a horizontal. The arrangement of the target points was varied relatively to the starting spot: Either one or two target points were displayed on the left or right side (same side) or one point was presented on each side of the currently fixated spot (different sides). All of the spots lay on the same horizontal and distances were held constant. What Findlay found, using the one target conditions as the referential baseline, was that the saccades' landing positions were biased towards the second target: They occurred to land between the two target spots in the conditions in which they appeared on the same side of the initial fixation. In the 'different sides' condition the magnitude of saccades was not affected; subjects saccaded precisely to either one or the other target. Interestingly, the latter condition produced an increase in mean saccadic latency, which could not be found in any of the other conditions.

In another experiment conducted by Findlay (1982), he examined if varied target characteristics and the subject's task influence the global effect. Eight different target configurations varying in number (one or two targets), size (small or big), equality (same size or different size) and eccentricity (5° or 10°) were shown to the subjects in two tasks. They were asked either to detect, if one of the squares is split in two halves indicated by a small gap or to compare if the currently presented arrangement of targets was the same as in the previous trial. In general, saccades were again made to intermediate spots between targets when a two-target arrangement was presented. For two visible targets of different sizes, the mean saccadic landing position was closer to the bigger of the two targets. When the targets were the same size, saccades landed closer to the nearer target. Consequently, the global effect can be influenced by characteristics of the target configuration.

Besides investigations on the impact of stimulus feature manipulations in the theoretical framework of the visual COG effect, there has also been research on top-down processes that might influence the discrepancy in saccadic landing positions.

For instance, Coëffé and O'Regan (1987) were able to show that the visual COG effect can also be influenced by the predictability of target location. Strings of nine letters were presented to the subjects varying the target position within the string. The subjects were asked to make saccades to the target letter indicated by crosses. The predictability of the target location was varied by presenting blocks in which the target location remained the same across trials (high predictability) and blocks in which the target location differed between trials (low predictability). The control condition, in which the target letter was presented alone, was also presented in high and low predictability blocks.

Accurate landing positions on the target were found when target letters were presented isolated. In the actual experimental condition, according to the authors the saccadic landing positions should have been biased towards the center of the string, which was between the fourth and fifth letter. As expected, saccades were overshooting targets presented on the second position in the letter string and undershooting targets presented on sixth or eighth position. Contrary results were found for saccades towards targets presented on the fourth position in the string: an overshoot was expected, but instead results yielded an undershoot of saccades for this case. That is why Coëffé and O'Regan (1987, p. 231) discussed a 'gaze attraction position', which was not equal to their initial definition of the COG. Plotting the saccadic landing position as a function of target location in string, they showed that the accurate landing position would have been theoretically around the third letter in string (cf. Figure 3a in Coëffé & O'Regan, 1987). That is why they suggested that a weighted average in the computation of the COG might be more accurate in predicting saccadic ending positions. For their results, a model that adds more weight to less eccentric objects than to objects in the further periphery seemed reasonable. However, as described above, McGowan et al. (1998) could not find a benefit for eccentricity dependent weighting.

More importantly, Coëffé and O'Regan's (1987) results yielded that these biases were stronger for the low predictability blocks, but also apparent in high predictability blocks. This shows that information about the position of non-target

37

objects influences gaze even if the subject is able to anticipate the correct position of the target. However, higher accuracy of saccadic landing positions in the latter case suggested that top-down process like predictability can indeed influence the visual COG effect.

In a subsequent experiment using the same experimental set-up and same conditions, they tested if the variation of saccadic latency influences saccadic accuracy. Indicating the start of a fixation by the disappearance of the fixation cross, saccadic latency was varied between blocks. The accuracy of saccadic landing was improved by increasing minimum saccade latency, while no effect of latency on accuracy was found in the control condition (Coëffé & O'Regan, 1987).

Up to this point, the majority of experiments on the visual COG effect used classical stimuli and tasks of vision research, since they work very well to investigate circumscribed aspects of visual phenomena. However, having considered the role of gaze in everyday life in section 1.3. *The Allocation of Gaze in Natural Tasks*, at least some results on the visual COG effect, that were found in experiments using more naturalistic stimuli and/or tasks, will be described in the following.

Vishwanath and Kowler (2003) were able to show that saccades to spatially extended objects – which are more common in reality – landed close to the visual COG of the object as a considered default reference position for saccades. In their experiment, they tested subjects in three different conditions. First, a single saccade task, in which the subjects were instructed to make only one saccade from the fixation point to the target, to look at the target 'as a whole' and to suppress further correction saccades. Second, the subjects were asked to make two or more saccades to and on the object to find their preferred spot to view the target 'as a whole'. Third, subjects had to do a more naturalistic task, particularly a sequential fixation task, making saccades between stimuli in a given sequence.

For all three conditions, the averaged saccadic landing position was close to the visual COG, even though the COG was outside the actual target stimulus due the shape of the used stimuli (angular versions of the letters 'O', 'C' and 'L' in different orientations). Most intriguingly, saccades were directed closest to the visual COG in the sequential fixation task, suggesting that the visual COG (mostly independent of other visual stimuli characteristics) is used as reference position in naturalistic tasks.

In another study by Vishwanath and Kowler, conducted in 2004, they further examined the influence of more naturalistic set-ups on the visual COG effect. In a series of experiments they, again, investigated the saccadic landing position in sequences of four saccades (similar to Vishwanath & Kowler, 2003), but besides using 2-D extended objects, they also built set-ups with 3-dimensional objects. They assumed that if depth information were not used for the control of saccades, then the landing position of saccades towards a 3-D target should land closely to the visual COG of their 2-D version (Vishwanath & Kowler, 2004).

By comparing the visual COG effects, they found that when 2-D objects were presented, subjects directed their gaze near the 2-D COG, which was specified as the centroid of the stimulus' density distribution. Results for 3-D objects and the 3-D COG that was set to the centroid of the stimulus' density distribution adjusted for depth looked different: One subject showed saccadic landing positions close to the 3-D COG for 3-D stimuli or between the 2-D and the 3-D COG. The second subject's saccades seemed to be even more biased by depth: The mean landing position was shifted away from the 3-D COG to the object's back edge (Vishwanath & Kowler, 2004).

To explain the differences between the 2-D and the 3-D objects they discussed a 'distance-scaled averaging model' for the 3-D stimuli, in which the control of saccadic landing positions is a "weighted average over the 2D image, where more weight is assigned to the portions projected to be further in depth" (Vishwanath & Kowler, 2004, p. 455). However, the results varied across subjects even in a retest of the results with a larger sample of five participants.

In sum, all these results demonstrate several important aspects with regard to the present study. First, they point out that information from the peripheral visual field does indeed influence where subjects look, in a variety of experimental set-ups involving different kinds of more or less naturalistic stimuli and tasks. The universality of the visual COG effect, was further demonstrated by studies that showed that this effect also occurs in reading (Vitu, 1991).

Secondly, they show that the visual COG occurs for both extended target configurations (Findlay, 1982; Vishwanath & Kowler, 2003) and for non-target distractors (Coren & Hoenig, 1972), which is interesting in terms of task relevance of the presented stimuli (see section 2.3. Stimuli and Task).

Admittedly, the concept itself is vague and the dissent about the actual crucial factors in the specification of the visual COG is not eliminated yet. Nevertheless, the influence of peripheral information that is depicted by the visual COG effect cannot be denied. As Morgan, Hole, and Glennerster (1990) stated, the extraction of a visual scene's centroid happens automatically while locating objects within it and therefore cannot be avoided. Under which circumstances it is used in the planning of saccades is another question.

Often referred to as saccadic landing *error* due to missing suppression of non-relevant visual information (Zhao, Gersch, Schnitzer, Dosher, & Kowler, 2012), the visual COG effect also offers less pessimistic interpretations than being a deficiency in the planning of saccades. For instance, already Findlay (1982) claimed the 'global effect' – how he termed the visual COG effect – can be viewed as a strategy to get as much information as possible from the target configuration. Morgan et al. (1990) further underlined the importance of locating objects for the purpose of interacting with one's environment in everyday life and that this ability is essential in both foveal and peripheral vision. Speaking of everyday life, until now only few studies have tested to what extent the visual COG effect occurs in natural settings (Vishwanath & Kowler, 2004). Possible influential variables might be features of the visual scene, like less uniformity than experimental stimuli (Vishwanath & Kowler, 2004); top-down processes, such as the cognitive goal of the agent; or simply the fact that the person is able to make head movements instead of making saccades while the head is fixed.

This understanding of the concept by Findlay (1982) and Morgan et al. (1990) was adopted herein. The next section will elaborate this idea by introducing the paradigm that has been the basis of the present study.

1.5. The Paradigm and the Aim of the Study

To examine if peripheral information can also influence the gaze position in naturalistic tasks, a VR experiment was conducted. Here, it is assumed that paying attention to several different task-relevant objects at the same time, leads to a tendency to fixate an intermediate spatial spot by which the person can get *maximal* information of the potentially important parts the current scene provides. This is contrary to the 'non-compromise gaze' assumption of the Walter model. However, as pointed out before, predicting human gaze allocation in natural tasks without considering the influence of peripheral vision is a simplification that is questioned herein.

In terms of foveal and peripheral vision, the maximization of information gathering can be viewed as an inevitable trade-off. Figure 1 illustrates this idea.

In the first case (see Figure 1A), fixating an object at its center provides high-quality information (according visual acuity) about this object. The trade-off here is that information about other objects in the further peripheral field might get lost completely.

In the second case (see Figure 1B), one can still acquire high-quality information about an object by fixating a spot on the object's edge. In addition, it is possible to get a fair amount of information about other objects, which might be visible in the peripheral field.

In the third case (see Figure 1C), directing gaze on an intermediate spot (between objects) does not yield valuable high-quality information from the fovea. However, one is able to receive quite a lot information about several objects in the closer periphery. The quality of this information is less accurate due to the decline of visual acuity.

Having these ideas in mind, the following questions will be addressed in the current study: How does peripheral information influence where we look? Do objects other than the currently fixated object influence the position of gaze? Can a gaze bias towards objects in the peripheral field (cf. visual COG effect in section 1.4. An Effect of Peripheral Information on Gaze) be shown in naturalistic tasks as conducted in VR? And further, is this gaze bias influenced by the current behavioral goal as the Walter model (Sprague et al., 2007) would predict?

41

The goal of the study is to provide a first attempt that the contribution of peripheral information should be considered in models of human visuomotor behavior, such as the Walter model. Experiments investigating the visual COG suggest that peripheral information can influence the allocation of gaze. Although, this effect is often interpreted as being a saccadic landing *error*, here, it is assumed that this bias can be advantageous in natural tasks by providing more possibly important information for the state estimate (see Figure 1).

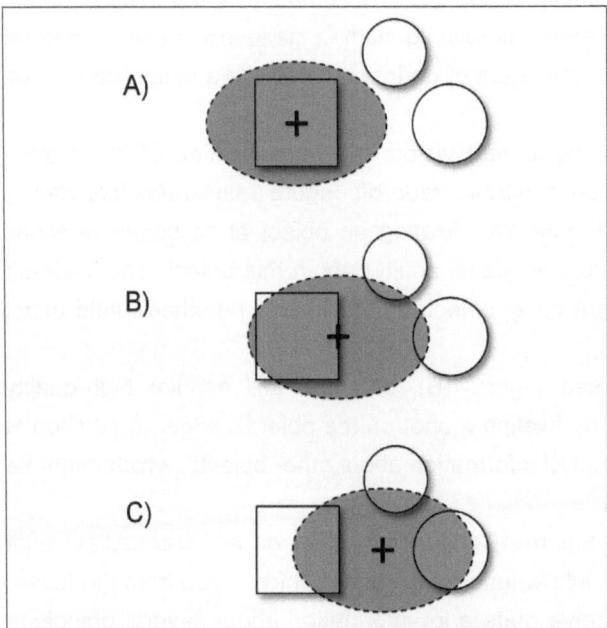

Figure 1. Illustration of three different gaze positions (black cross) in the same scene showing three objects (square and circles). The visual field of the observer is shown by the dashed outlined grey area.

Consequently, a visual COG effect in a naturalistic environment is expected. Moreover, hand in hand with the Walter model, this bias should be influenced by the current task. If this can be shown, the simplification of predicting where a person will look next by only using parameters of the current foveal image should be reconsidered.

The next section will state the hypotheses of the present study more specifically.

1.6. Hypotheses and Implementation

Following the questions raised in the previous section, the hypotheses investigated in the previous study are as follows:

First, current information from the peripheral visual field does influence gaze position, that is, there is a gaze bias towards other objects, which are visible in the periphery. In particular, fixations biased *towards* neighboring objects should be more frequent than fixations biased in the opposite direction.

Second, this tendency is modulated by the current task, respectively, by the ensuing implicit reward of achieving the goal of the task. That means that the gaze bias towards peripheral objects (first hypothesis) appears more frequently when these objects are relevant to the current task than when they are not. Namely, the gaze bias towards targets happens more frequently when the task is to collect targets, while the gaze bias towards obstacles is shown more often when the current task asks to avoid obstacles.

The examination of these hypotheses was conducted in a virtual environment set-up using eye and body tracking equipment to collect eye movement data while subjects walked through a virtual laboratory. The task-relevance of visible objects was varied by different task instructions (*collect targets* vs. *avoid obstacles* vs. *both tasks at once*) on the one hand and by presenting objects of two different colors indicating targets and obstacles (or respectively neutral objects, depending on task) on the other hand. The gaze data were subdivided into single fixations and categorized by the object (target or obstacle), that was currently fixated. The relative frequencies of fixations were analyzed to see if the positions of neighboring objects and their task-relevance produced differences. Further specifications on procedure and methods are given in the following chapter.

2. Methods

This second section will give details on how the virtual environment was built up and how eye movement data were collected. It will further give a description of what the virtual room looked like and what the subjects had to do to accomplish the given tasks. Additionally, it will outline the experimental design and the procedure. First, the sample of participants is described.

2.1. Sample

Twelve subjects participated in the present experiment. The six males and six females were on average M = 19 years old (Min = 18, Max = 26). All of them had normal or corrected-to-normal vision by contact lenses. Persons wearing glasses were excluded from participation beforehand. Ten subjects were college freshmen at The University of Texas at Austin and were paid in participation hours, which they had to collect as credits for their psychology class. The two remaining subjects (one graduate student and one research associate) participated voluntarily. All participants, except for the research associate – whose data did not differ profoundly from those of the other participants' – were naïve about the research question and had no experience with virtual reality experiments.

2.2. Equipment

The experiment took place in a laboratory at The University of Texas at Austin. Customary computers were used for programming the experiment as well as for conducting, storing, and analyzing the data.

For the construction of the interactive virtual environment and for rendering the graphics throughout the experiment, the Vizard Virtual Reality Software Toolkit by Worldviz®was used.

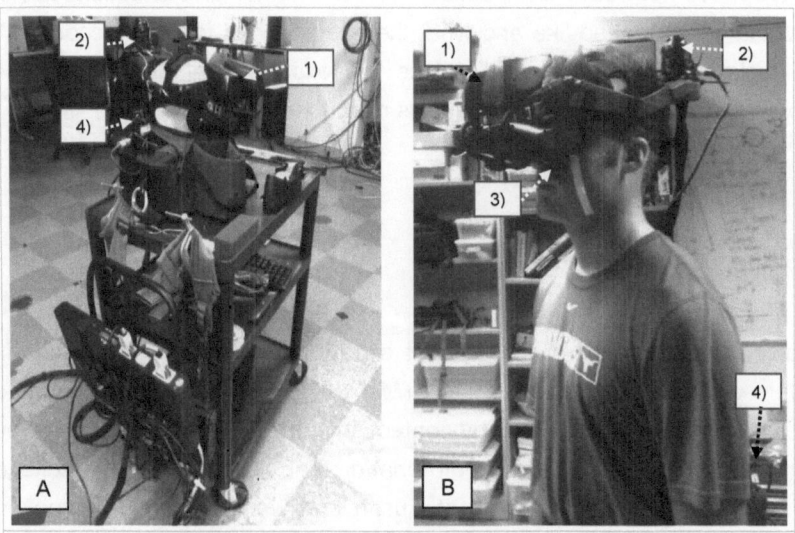

Figure 2. A) The technical equipment used in the present experiment and B) subject EM wearing it. 1) The two screens of the nVisor SX111 wide field-of-view head-mounted display, giving the subject an impression of a 3-D image. 2) One HiBALL™-3100 Tracker (head position) attached to the backside of the head mount. 3) The camera of the View Point Eye Tracker® below the subject's left eye. 4) The second HiBALL™-3100 Tracker (body position) put into a belt bag (blue in A), which the subject wore around the waist.

To enable the participants to freely move through the virtual environment, the subjects wore an nVisor SX111 wide field-of-view head-mounted display by NVIS Inc. (resolution: 1280x1024pixel; spatial resolution: 3.6arc-min/pixel; contrast: >

100:1; total horizontal FOV: 102°; total vertical FOV: 64°; overlap: 50° ≙ 66%). It compassed two screens (one for each eye) to create the impression of a 3-dimensional image (see Figure 2). Attached to the backside of this helmet was one of two HiBALL™-3100 Tracker by 3rdTech™ to record the subject's head movements (i.e. turning to the left or right). The second HiBALL™-3100 Tracker was put into a belt bag, which the subject wore around the waist, recording the subject's movements through the room. Both trackers are necessary to align the subject's actions and the rendering of the current image, and therefore, to allow the subject to interact with the virtual environment.

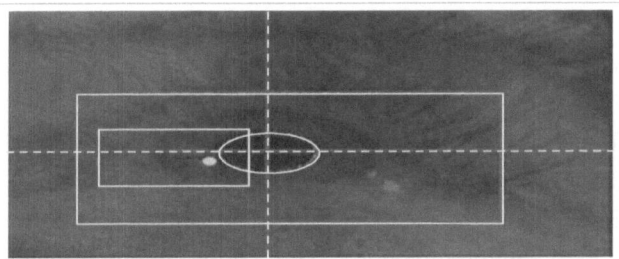

Figure 3. View of the eye tracking camera on the subject's left eye. The eye tracking software calculated the gaze position by using the pupil-glint vector. The bigger white box marks the area in which the pupil should be detectable; the smaller white box marks the area in which the glint (= cornea reflection of an infrared light attached to the eye tracking camera; represented by small white spot) should be detectable. The bigger circle indicates size and movement of the pupil. From these parameters results an estimation of gaze location shown by the white cross-hairs (dashed lines), respectively by those in Figure 7.

The optical sensors of the HiBALL™-3100 Tracker are 7.3cm tall (5.4cm in diameter) and consist of six lenses and photodiodes. They have a maximum update rate of 1000Hz each (resolution of position: 0.2mm RMS; resolution of orientation: 0.01° RMS) with a latency of less than 1msec. Using infrared signals the sensors communicate with about 3000 infrared LEDs attached to the ceiling to cover the area of the laboratory, which the subjects could freely walk through. Eye movements of the left eye were recorded with a View Point Eye Tracker® by Arrington Research, Inc. The provided calibration software was adapted to in-house requirements, which resulted in a nine-point calibration screen. The pupil-glint vector was used as a reliable measure of eye movements (see Figure 3).

Auditory feedback when subjects made contact with a virtual object was given via customary speakers.

Eye movement data and video sequences from the subject's point of view during the experiment was stored and analyzed off line.

2.3. Stimuli and Task

The environment used in this study was a virtual replica of the actual real-world laboratory in which the experiment took place. The size of the virtual room was 7.3 x 7.9 meters and had comparable objects, such as desks and shelves, standing on the wall (see Figure 4).

The path, on which the subjects were instructed to stay on during the trials, was indicated by a light grey diagonal on the floor (length: 6.1 meters, width: 1.5 meters) between two opposite corners of the room (see Figure 5). A virtual elevator, which took the subjects up to the next room, was displayed by a green disk at the end of each path.

Arranged along the path were pink and blue cubes (size: $0.23m^3$). From now on, these cubes will be referred to as *objects*; other visible objects, for instance desks on the wall or the elevator disk on the floor, are interpreted as being part of the room, because they were not relevant to the subject's task and therefore not included when talking about objects. The cubes were stationary, hanging in the air and adjusted to the subject's individual eye height (about 0.5-0.6 feet less than subject's body height).

The subject's task was to collect and/or avoid objects of a certain color as instructed before each block of trials. They were told by one of the examiners, if they were about to collect blue or pink targets, to avoid blue or pink obstacles or to collect the one *while* avoiding the other color. The color, representing the type and task relevance of an object, remained the same within a subject, but was balanced across subjects.

48

To collect an object the subject had to walk through it until it disappeared. As point of reference served the HIBALL™-3100 Tracker, which the subject was wearing on the backside. More precisely, the body tracker's coordinates were shifted 0.4 meters forward to represent the subject's horizontal center of body. Thus, when the subject's body coordinates and the object coordinates were aligned (range: +/- 0.381 meters) the system recognized the object as being contacted by the subject and the object disappeared. Additionally, whenever subjects made contact with an object they heard an acoustic feedback: a fanfare, when collecting a task-relevant target; a buzzer sound when accidentally making contact with a task-relevant obstacle; or a bubble pop when walking through a task-irrelevant cube of either color.

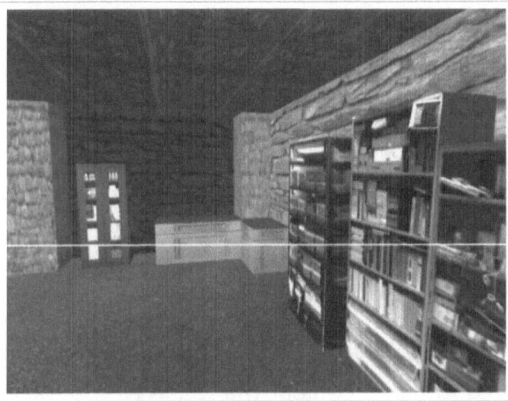

Figure 4. The view into the virtual laboratory, with desks (wooden ashlars in the back right corner), cupboards (upright block on the back wall), and shelves (on the right wall). The furniture was sited to the positions of the actual furniture in the real laboratory.

The idea of giving an acoustic feedback was to remind the subjects of the type of objects and the task they were doing in the experimental trials. More important than that was to reinforce the subject according to the implicit reward approach: A cheerful fanfare sound as a positive feedback when collecting a target; an unpleasant buzzer sound when making contact with an obstacle they should have had avoided; or a neutral bubble pop when the object was not task-relevant in this particular block of trials.

49

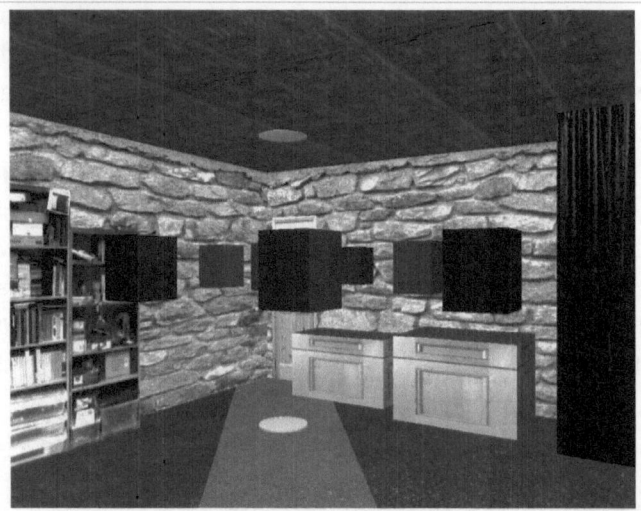

Figure 5. The viewpoint of the subject when arriving in the room via the elevator in the back corner. Virtual simulations of the real furniture are visible on the walls. The path the subjects had to stay on during the trial is indicated by a light grey strip on the floor; the elevator to the next room is indicated by the disks. The cubes (originally pink and cyan) were adjusted to the subject's individual eye height and the subject was instructed beforehand which color represented a target and which represented an obstacle, respectively, which ones were relevant in the current task.

These sounds were learned by the subjects in a practice room before each block, in which they were told to make contact with each type of object. This practice room was also the virtual replica of the laboratory, but did not have the grey path on the floor and the objects were distributed randomly across the whole room.

2.4. Design

The total number of objects arranged along the path varied between 6, 8, 10, 12, or 14 objects in total. The division of the two colors was kept constantly on 50%

cyan and 50% pink objects throughout the trials. For each number of objects, two rooms with different collocations of the objects were designed, which results in ten different rooms that were used for each task in random order. In this randomization, the direction was held constant, that means for each number of objects the subjects started one room in corner A and the other one in corner B.

To control for salience effects and implicitly existing interpretation of the two colors (e.g. reddish means danger), their meaning regarding the type of object (target vs. obstacle) was balanced across subjects (manipulated by verbal instructions): Half of the subjects faced pink targets and blue obstacles while the other half faced blue targets and pink obstacles.

Also balanced across subjects was the order of the three tasks to avoid order effects: Half of the sample started with the collecting targets (CT) task, while the other half started with the avoiding obstacles (AO) task. For both groups, the task in which they had to do both tasks at once (BOTH) was always the last one.

In total, each subject ran 30 trials: Ten for each task in three consecutive blocks separated by the practice room for each task.

Balancing the meaning of the two colors (pink targets and blue obstacles vs. blue targets and pink obstacles) and the order of the task (CT, AO, BOTH vs. AO, CT, BOTH) resulted in four different groups to which the subjects were assigned randomly, so that three subjects were in each group.

Emerging from the methods described above, the data analysis considered three within-subject factors: (a) The *Task* which the subjects had to accomplish, namely collecting targets (CT), avoiding obstacles (AO) or collecting targets while avoiding obstacles (BOTH); (b) The *Type of Fixated Object*, either target or obstacle; and (c) the *Type of Neighbor*, target or obstacle. The ensuing 3*2*2 design was completely crossed, but since fixations depended on the subjects' behavior (i.e. where they were looking) the number of situations for each combination of factor levels has not been balanced (see section 3. Results).

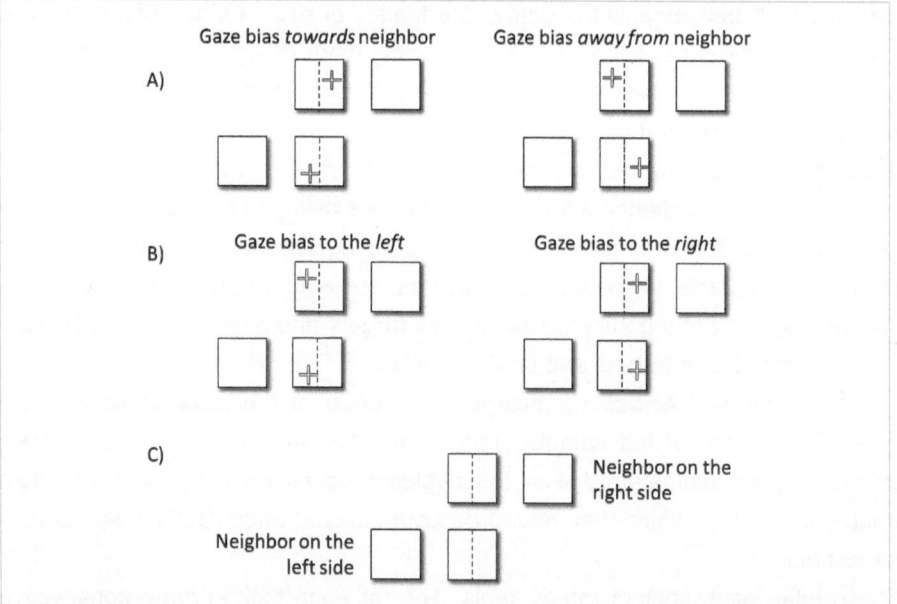

Figure 6. Illustration of the dependent variable (A) and the two confounding variables (B and C). A) On the left side, two situations are depicted in which the gaze position (cross) is biased in the same direction, in which the neighbor was present. Whereas on the right side, two situations are shown, in which gaze is biased in the opposite direction. B) The two figures on the left demonstrate a gaze preference towards the left side of the fixated objects, independent of the position of the neighbor. Analogously, the figures on the right show a gaze tendency towards the right side of the fixated object independent of the neighbor's position. C) The lowest figure simply depicts the two situations of object configuration regardless of relative fixation position: The neighbor can be either on the right or on the left side of the fixated object (= cube with dashed line indicating the center).

The dependent variable, used here to examine the expected gaze bias (for details on research questions see section 1.6. Hypotheses and Implementation) was the frequency of how often the subjects were fixating on an object with a tendency either *towards* or *away from* the neighboring object. Figure 6A illustrates these two cases for situations in which two objects were present in the subject's visual field. Fixations on an object were counted as 'biased towards neighbor', (a) if the neighbor was visible on the right side of the fixated object *and* the gaze position was on the right side of the center of the fixated object or (b) if the neighbor was visible on the left side of the fixated object *and* the gaze position was on the left side of the center of the fixated object. Fixations 'biased away from the neighbor' were defined as gaze positions being on the right side of the center of the fixated object while the second object was present on the left side of the fixated object or vice versa.

2.5. Procedure

The next two paragraphs will provide a description on how the experiment was conducted as a whole (see section 2.5.1. Procedure of the Experimental Conduct) and what a single trial looked like (see section 2.5.2. Procedure of a Trial).

2.5.1. Procedure of the Experimental Conduct

At first, the participants signed a general informed consent form (approved by the Institutional Review Board of the University of Texas at Austin) on participating, possible risks, and their rights and they completed a short demographic questionnaire. Then, they were verbally briefed about the used equipment, the procedure of the experiment, and their task (see Appendix A[1]) by one of the examiners. Nevertheless, the subjects remained naïve about the research questions until after the experiment.

Several arrangements needed to be made for each subject before the experiment could be carried out. First, the head-mounted displays and the position of the eye tracking camera needed to be adjusted to the participant's head, so that the camera could get a good track of the subject's eye, but did not block the subject's view on the two displays. Second, the subject buckled on a

---

[1] The appendix is available on the book's product page on www.springer.com.

belt bag around the waist carrying the second body tracker on the back. Third, the height of the virtual cubes was aligned to the participant's individual eye height. Last, the eye tracker was calibrated using Viewpoint® software (see section 2.2. Equipment).

Throughout the experiment, two examiners were present in the laboratory. One read a set of standardized instructions (see Appendix A) to the subjects before the experiment and gave further instructions about the subsequent task in the practice rooms. In addition, this examiner followed the subject through the laboratory making sure the subject did not run into real-world objects, such as cords for example. The other examiner was keeping track of the subject's eye movements and calibration accuracy during the experiment.

The experiment was conducted in three consecutive blocks, one for each task, consisting of ten trials with one preceding practice trial. This practice room contained randomly arranged objects of both colors. Participants were instructed verbally about the subsequent task and were given time to familiarize with the virtual room and what it feels, sounds, and looks like when making contact with the cubes by walking through them. Besides that, they heard the sounds when making contact with the objects depending on the task of the subsequent block. For instance, assuming the subject was confronted with pink targets and cyan obstacles and the subsequent task was to avoid obstacles: The subject got the instruction to avoid the cyan obstacles in the following block and that the pink cubes were not task-relevant. That means, it made no difference for the accomplishment of task, if the pink cubes were contacted or not. Then, the subject was asked to walk around the practice room and to make randomly contact with objects of both colors. When the subject walked through a task-relevant obstacle, an unpleasant buzzer sound was played via speakers. When the subject walked through a not task-relevant pink cube, a neutral bubble pop was audible.

Once the subject felt comfortable enough in the virtual environment and was familiar with the task, the subject was allowed to step on the green elevator disk to get to the next room and start the actual experimental trials.

The accuracy of the eye tracker was checked and calibration was renewed if necessary at the beginning, between blocks, and at the end of the experiment.

54

After all 30 trials had been completed, the subject was debriefed regarding the particular research question and was paid for the participation. In total, the experiment took 30 minutes to 1 hour for each participant, depending on the time needed for calibration and the subject's individual walking speed.

2.5.2. Procedure of a Trial

From the perspective of the participant, a single trial within the experiment looked as follows.

The subjects arrived in the virtual room in one of the two corners by the virtual elevator. Since the walls of the elevator were partly transparent, subjects were able to see the virtual room and the contained objects before the elevator got inactive and they were allowed to start walking. Instructed to stay on the greyish path and to walk as naturally as possible, subjects started to cross the room towards the opposite corner. While walking they were performing one of the three tasks (collect targets, avoid obstacles or both at the same time) as instructed before the block. After arriving at the opposite corner, the subjects had to step on the green elevator disk, which took them up to the next room and the next trial.

2.6. Data Preparation and Handcoding

To make the collected data usable for present calculations, first, an algorithm developed in-house was employed to compute when and where subjects were making fixations. The deduction of this kind of data was made possible by extracting and factoring in (a) recorded information about the subject's actions by the eye, body and head tracker, (b) the recorded video data of what the subject was seeing, and (c) the information about the objects' positions in the configuration files used to create the virtual environment.

Certain criteria were used by this 'fixation finder' algorithm to define a cluster of gaze positions as being one fixation; importantly for reasons of smoothing single outliers, the median of positions across three frames (reference frame +/- 1) was assigned. First, the velocity of the eye movements had to be below 60°/sec to be rated as a steady fixation. Second, to avoid a great quantity of very short fixations, they had to last at least 80msec. Third, if two fixation clusters were separated by a blink shorter than 80msec and the distance between positions of gaze before and after the blink was not greater than 1°, they were aggregated to one single fixation.

In another step, each fixation was labeled, if it has been upon a target, upon an obstacle or not upon an object. To do this, each data frame was reconstructed by the algorithm to figure out if and which kind of object was present at the location of the fovea (circular area around the actual fixation point, 30pixel in diameter). The fixation was labeled after the present object, when most of its frames (see step before) were spent on this object. Due to inevitable inaccuracies in measurements of eye movements, the size of this 'virtual fovea' was chosen to be 30pixel, so that gaze positions that were close to an object were labeled to be *on* the particular object as well.

Next, four observers (the author and three associates) reclassified the fixations found by the algorithm by watching the subjects' video sequences frame by frame. These video sequences contained a record of what the subjects saw during the experiment superimposed by a cross-hairs representing the estimate of the gaze position provided by the eye tracker. The observers were briefed about the research question and the handcoding criteria (as follows below). One practice file was watched and handcoded by all of them to check for comprehension of the criteria and the alignment between observers.

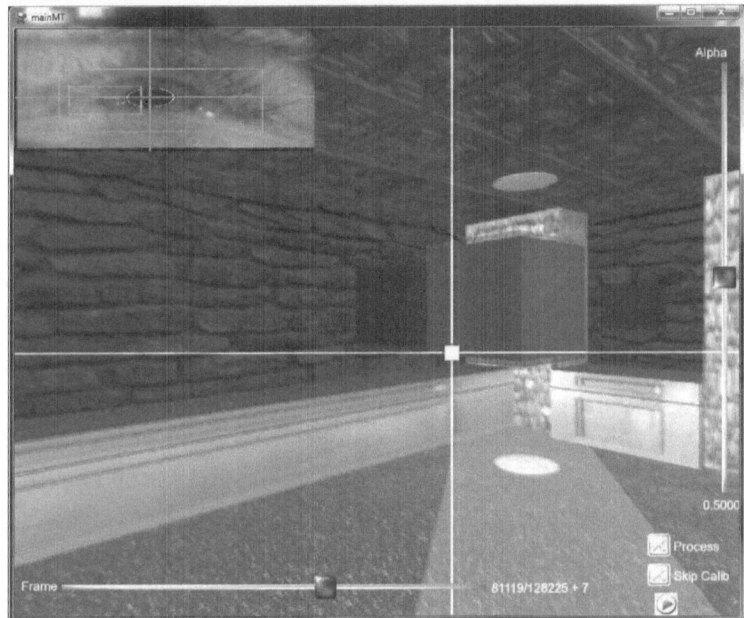

Figure 7. The viewpoint of the subject while walking along the path. The white superimposed cross-hairs and the small white box indicate where the subject was directing the center of gaze. In the upper left corner, the subject's left eye is visible for the examiner. To make the process of handcoding a little more comprehensible, the pictured scene serves as an example (assuming currently fixated cube was an obstacle and the two darker cubes were targets): In this case, the observer would have noted that an obstacle was fixated and that two targets were visible in the periphery. In addition, the examiner would have annotated the positions of gaze and the objects by clicking on the center of gaze (white box) and the two-dimensional centers of the cubes.

For reasons of simplicity, only fixations, during which one to four objects were present in the subject's visual field, were considered. Fixations made in the practice rooms and while taking the elevator were excluded, as were fixations upon the green elevator disk. Of the remaining fixations, the observers noted the types of the visible objects (target vs. obstacle) and the *horizontal* position (i.e. the x coordinates) of both the centers of visible objects and the fixation cross by using an in-house built software add-on. For an example, see Figure 7.

Besides the exclusion criteria mentioned above, fixations found by the algorithm were excluded, if they seemed problematic in the eye of the observer. For instance, if the eye tracker lost track of the subject's pupil or glint (see upper left corner of Figure 7) or if the majority of frames of a particular fixation were not *on* a target or an obstacle (e.g. if a fixated target was collected during the fixation and the remaining frames were on the wall or object behind it).

From the annotated horizontal positions of fixations and object centers, the relative horizontal positions were calculated using MATLAB™. The reference point here was the center of the fixated object. Thus, the positions of fixations were categorized as being left or right of the object center and the neighboring objects were categorized, as either left or right of the center of the fixated object. The categorization was held dichotomously since borders of a middle category for fixations around the object center would have had to be arbitrarily chosen due to varying viewing angles.

All further analyses were conducted using IBM® SPSS Statistics 18. Their results are presented in the following chapter.

3. Results

This section will describe the analyses and all results of the data obtained from the previously described data collection. First, absolute numbers of fixations will be reported and reasons for excluded data will be given (see section 3.1. Total Frequencies of Fixations and Exclusion of Data). Secondly, results to answer the research questions raised above will be presented (see section 3.2. The Gaze Bias Towards Neighbors for Two Visible Objects). Last, further factors that might interfere with the results will be analyzed to rule out possible confounding effects (see section 3.3. Screening of Possibly Interfering Direction Effects).

3.1. Total Frequencies of Fixations and Exclusion of Data

The total number of fixations found by the fixation finder algorithm was $M = 2113$ ($SD = 310$) on average for each subject (see Appendix B, Table B1 for more detailed information), of which, only $M = 825$ fixations ($SD = 211$) per subject were automatically categorized to be on objects (i.e. targets, obstacles, elevator). Of this population, fixations were excluded by hand due to two reasons: (a) they did not meet the observers' quality requirements or (b) they were made in non-experimental trials. This process left about $M= 238$ fixations ($SD = 76$) per subject. That is, an exclusion of 71.2% due to the exclusion criteria described in section 2.6. *Data Preparation and Handcoding*.

After this first data preparation, the fixation situations, in which three or four objects were visible, were excluded from further analyses due to small numbers of occurrence (see Appendix B, Table B1). Admittedly, the total numbers of fixations were not much lower than for one or two objects, but with a growing number of neighbors, the number of factors increases as well. This resulted in very small numbers of fixations for the single combinations of factor levels.

Thus, of the remaining valid 2859 fixations (M = 238 fixations, SD = 76) after handcoding, only the data of fixations with two visible objects were analyzed, that is a total number of 766 fixations with an average of M = 64 fixations per subject (SD = 30). Consequently, the analyzed data represent about 27% of the total data after handcoding. For more detailed information about the number of fixations made by each subject, see Appendix Table B2.

As becomes apparent by looking at Table 1, across all tasks the number of fixations on obstacles was relatively small, namely less than one sixth of the number of fixations on targets. This suggests that subjects showed a general preference to look at targets (independent of the target's current task-relevance).

Table 1. The absolute frequencies of fixations and marginal sums across subjects (N = 12) and across tasks for the combinations of Type of Fixated Object and Type of Neighbor.

Overall		Type of **Neighbor**		
		Target	Obstacle	
Type of **Fixated** Object	Target	210	451	661
	Obstacle	83	22	105
		293	473	766

Tables 2 to 4 show the total numbers of fixations for each category of factor level combination (3 Tasks * 2 Types of Fixated Object * 2 Types of Neighbor). In all three tasks, the number of fixations on obstacles was small, especially when a second obstacle was present in the periphery.

Another important fact to mention here is the small number of fixations in the AO task compared to the remaining two tasks with comparable total numbers. Even while conducting the experiment and during the handcoding process, it grew apparent that some subjects did not make any fixations on objects in some trials of the AO task. Sometimes, fixations were only made between objects or on the path and the elevator.

Table 2. The absolute frequencies of fixations and marginal sums across subjects (N = 12) for the combinations of Type of Fixated Object and Type of Neighbor in the CT task.

Collect Targets		Type of Neighbor		
		Target	Obstacle	
Type of Fixated Object	Target	103	193	296
	Obstacle	33	6	39
		136	199	335

Table 3. The absolute frequencies of fixations and marginal sums across subjects (N = 12) for the combinations of Type of Fixated Object and Type of Neighbor in the AO task.

Avoid Obstacles		Type of Neighbor		
		Target	Obstacle	
Type of Fixated Object	Target	14	51	65
	Obstacle	14	11	25
		28	62	90

Table 4. The absolute frequencies of fixations and marginal sums across subjects (N = 12) for the combinations of Type of Fixated Object and Type of Neighbor in the BOTH task.

Both		Type of Neighbor		
		Target	Obstacle	
Type of Fixated Object	Target	93	207	300
	Obstacle	36	5	41
		129	212	341

After having reported the findings on the total numbers of fixations made by subjects, the subsequent section will present the results of the analyses conducted for testing the hypotheses (see section 1.6. Hypotheses and Implementation).

3.2. The Gaze Bias Towards Neighbors for Two Visible Objects

Before presenting the statistical results of the analysis (see 3.2.2. The Analysis of the Gaze Bias Towards Neighboring Objects), the dependent variable and its transformation to a normally distributed variable will be explained and justified in the following.

3.2.1. The Computation of a New Variable

For two visible objects, a new variable was computed using the horizontal gaze position relative to the center of the fixated object (left vs. right of object center) and the position of the second, not fixated object (from here on referred to as *neighbor*) relative to the fixated object (left vs. right of the latter). The new computed variable contains both pieces of information by distinguishing if the position of gaze had a tendency *towards* the neighboring object (*same direction*) or *away from* it (*opposite direction*). An illustrative example is given in Figure 6A.

The relative frequencies of fixations in the same direction as the neighbor were calculated for each subject and each combination of Task, Type of Fixated Object, and Type of Neighbor.

Because relative frequencies (h) do not meet the assumption of normal distribution, they needed to be transformed using an arcsine transformation (after Irtel, 2013)

$$h' = \cos^{-1}(\sqrt{h}) \qquad\qquad (1)$$

prior to the conduct of parametric tests.

For reasons of comprehensibility, the arcsine-transformed values were recalculated to relative frequencies ($0 \leq h \leq 1$) using the inverse function

$$h = (\sin(h'))^2 \qquad\qquad (2)$$

before reporting.

Therefore, results described in this section as well as the results displayed in Figures 8 to 19 show relative frequencies, while the tables in the appendix contain the analyzed arcsine transformed values before the recalculation.

Since relative frequencies were calculated for fixations, which were biased towards the neighbor opposed to fixations biased in the opposite direction, values above chance mean 'same direction', whereas values below chance stand for 'opposite direction'.

3.2.2. The Analysis of the Gaze Bias Towards Neighboring Objects

To begin with the least complex result, the overall mean of relative frequencies across all subjects, tasks and object types were calculated and tested against chance ($\alpha = 0.05$). As Figure 8 displays, the overall mean of relative frequencies of fixations that were biased towards the neighbor was $M = 0.726$ (*SEM* $= 0.022$) and with $t(11) = 9.57$, $p < .001$ significantly higher than chance, which indicates a general tendency to make fixations biased towards objects in the periphery (see Appendix B, Tables B3 and B4).

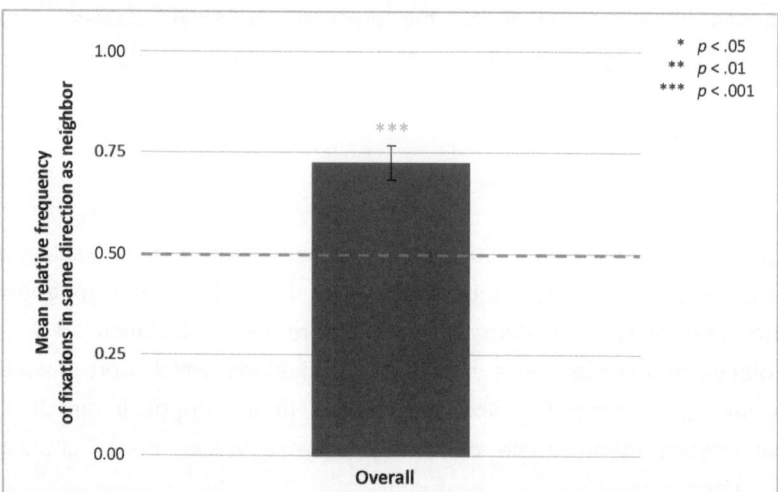

Figure 8. The overall mean of relative frequencies of fixations on an object biased towards a neighbor averaged across subjects (N = 12), tasks, object types and direction. Values above chance (dashed line) indicate a more frequent occurrence of fixations biased towards neighboring objects; values below indicate a more frequent occurrence of fixations biased in the opposite direction. Grey stars mark results of one sample t-tests against chance. Error bars represent the confidence interval of 95%.

To check if this general gaze bias towards neighbors is vindicated for objects on the left as well as objects on the right side of the fixated object, the analysis was repeated for the distinct directions with Bonferroni adjusted alpha of 2.5% (see Figure 9). The analysis revealed that in both cases fixations, biased towards the neighbor, were made more often than in the opposite direction (M_{Right} = 0.717, SEM_{Right} = 0.061; M_{Left} = 0.771, SEM_{Left} = 0.044; see Appendix B, Table B5). Both were significantly higher than chance, $t_{Right}(11)$ = 3.28, p = .007 and $t_{Left}(11)$ = 5.44, $p <$ .001 (see Appendix B, Table B6), but not significantly different from each other, $t(11)$ = -0.65, p = .529 (see Appendix B, Table B7). Thus, the gaze tendency towards objects other than the currently fixated one seems to be true and analogous for neighbors on the left and on the right side.

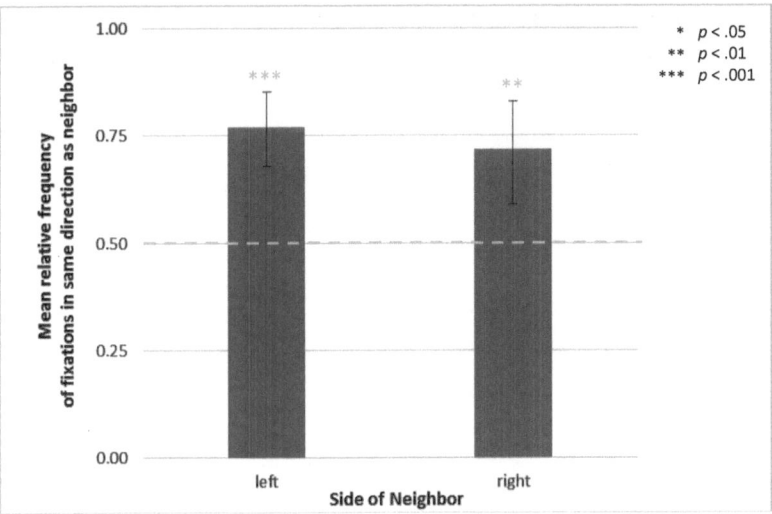

Figure 9. The means of relative frequencies of fixations on an object biased towards a neighbor averaged across subjects (N = 12), tasks and object types for situations, in which the neighbor was visible on the left or the right side (α adjusted after Bonferroni: α per test = 0.05/2= 0.025). For details on figure elements, see Figure 8.

A 3-way analysis of variance (ANOVA) was conducted for the three within-subject factors Task (CT, AO, BOTH), Type of Fixated Object (target, obstacle), and Type of Neighbor (target, obstacle) to examine if these factors produce differences in the mean arcsine-transformed relative frequencies of fixations biased towards the neighbor. In addition, paired samples t-tests have been conducted post-hoc to further compare significant effects. Above that, one sample t-tests were calculated to examine if the relative frequencies for fixations in the same direction as the neighbor were different from chance. For all analyses, alpha was set to 5%, adjusted after Bonferroni for the post-hoc t-tests.

For some combinations of factor levels (see Appendix B, Table B8), no fixations were handcoded for a couple of subjects (see Appendix B, Table B2, cells containing zeroes). Thus, the missing values needed to be substituted for further analysis. Since the relative frequencies for same and opposite direction sum up to 1, substituting the missing values by the arcsine-transformed chance level, which is roughly 0.785, seemed reasonably conservative. In total, 42 missing values (29.17%) needed to be substituted, more than half of them in the categories, in which two obstacles were visible.

Under given sphericity (see Appendix B, Table B9), the ANOVA revealed significant main effects for the Type of the Fixated Object, $F(1,11) = 16.56$, $p = .002$, and the Type of Neighbor, $F(1,11) = 7.45$, $p = .020$ (see Appendix B, Table B10).

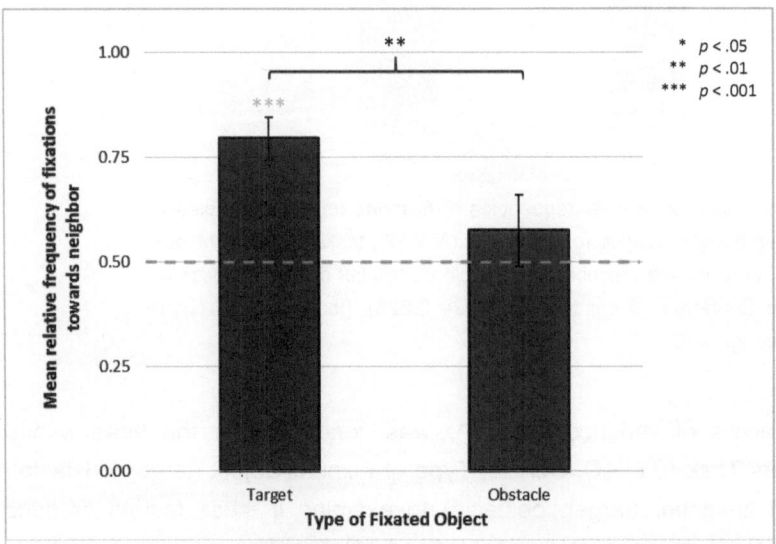

Figure 10. The means of relative frequencies ($N = 12$) of fixations on an object biased towards a neighbor for the different Types of the Fixated Object (target vs. obstacle). For details on figure elements, see Figure 8; black stars mark results of the 3-way ANOVA.

For the Type of Fixated Object, the gaze bias towards neighbors happened more often if a target was fixated than if an obstacle was fixated (see Figure 10 & Appendix B, Tables B11 and B12). Post-hoc t-tests showed that only if the fixated object was a target, the bias towards the neighbor was significantly different from chance ($M_{FixTarg} = 0.796$, $SEM_{FixTarg} = 0.026$, $t_{FixTarg}(11) = 9.85$, $p < .001$; $M_{FixObst} = 0.575$, $SEM_{FixObst} = 0.044$, $t_{FixObst}(11) = 1.70$, $p = .118$).

Similar results were obtained for the Type of Neighbor. When the neighbor was a target, subjects showed the gaze bias towards it more often than when it was a neighboring obstacle (see Figure 11 & Appendix B, Tables B13 and B14). In both cases, the effect was significantly greater than chance (M_{NbTarg} = 0.745, SEM_{NbTarg} = 0.029, $t_{NbTarg}(11)$ = 7.74, p < .001; M_{NbObst} = 0.635, SEM_{NbObst} = 0.032, $t_{NbObst}(11)$ = 4.08, p = .002).

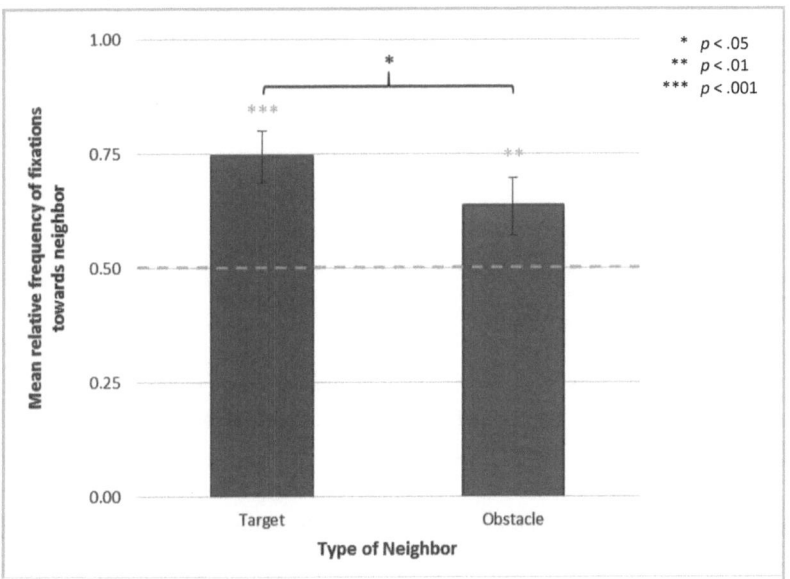

Figure 11. The means of relative frequencies (N = 12) of fixations on an object biased towards a neighbor for the different Types of Neighbor (target vs. obstacle). For details on figure elements, see Figure 8; black stars mark results of the 3-way ANOVA.

The factor Task, taken by itself, did not have a significant effect on gaze bias, $F_{Task}(2,22)$ = 0.24, p = .793 (see Figure 12 & Appendix B, Table B10). Albeit, there was no significant difference between tasks, the one sample t-tests showed that in all three of them the relative frequencies were significantly higher than chance (M_{CT} = 0.710, SEM_{CT} = 0.044; M_{AO} = 0.667, SEM_{AO} = 0.047; M_{BOTH} = 0.696, SEM_{BOTH} = 0.038; see Appendix B, Table B15). Hence, gaze was biased towards neighbors in all three conditions ($t_{CT}(11) = 4.40$, $p = .001$; $t_{AO}(11) = 3.41$, $p = .006$; $t_{BOTH}(11) = 4.85$, $p = .001$; see Appendix B, Table B16).

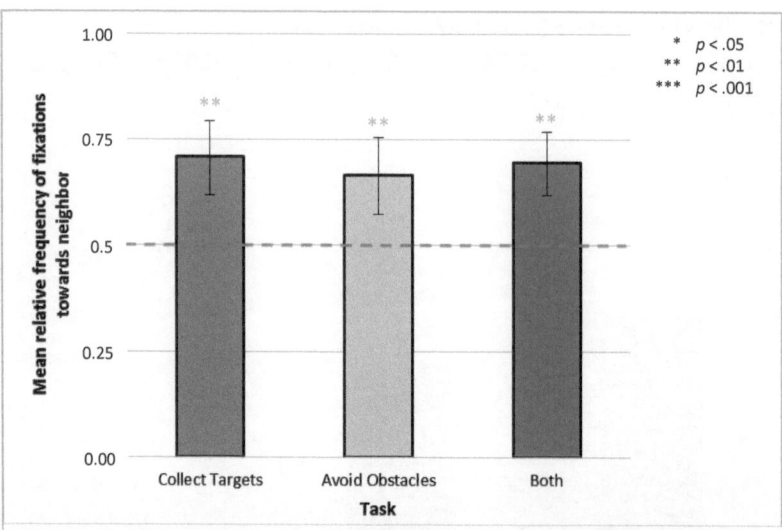

Figure 12. The means of relative frequencies ($N = 12$) of fixations on an object biased towards a neighbor for the three different Tasks (collect targets vs. avoid obstacles vs. both at once). For details on figure elements, see Figure 8.

Nevertheless, the interaction between Task and the Type of Neighbor was significant, $F_{Task*Nb}(2,22) = 3.76$, $p = .039$ (see Appendix B, Table B10). As can be seen in Figure 13, the means were higher than chance for all combinations of factor levels (see Appendix B, Table B17), but only significantly different from it for the following combination: CT*target ($t(11) = 3.57$, $p = .004$), CT*obstacle ($t(11) = 3.65$, $p = .004$), AO*obstacle ($t(11) = 2.90$, $p = .015$) and BOTH*target ($t(11) = 6.05$, $p < .001$; see Table 5 and Appendix B, Table B18).

Although the mean relative frequencies were not significantly different from chance for AO*target ($t(11) = 1.21$, $p = .253$) and BOTH*obstacle ($t(11) = 0.75$, $p = .467$), the data show that there is also a trend to make fixations biased towards neighbors.

68

Table 5. The means (and SEM) of relative frequencies (N = 12) of fixations on an object biased towards a neighbor for all combinations of the within-subject factors Task (collect targets, avoid obstacles, both at once) and Type of Neighbor (target, obstacle).

		Type of Neighbor	
		Target	Obstacle
Task	CT	0.777 (0.067)	0.639 (0.037)
	AO	0.611 (0.089)	0.721 (0.069)
	BOTH	0.832 (0.044)	0.539 (0.051)

By looking at Figure 13, it becomes apparent that the data show the same trend for the CT task and the BOTH task, revealing higher mean relative frequencies for neighboring targets than for neighboring obstacles. In the AO task, the results are vice versa, showing a higher mean for neighboring obstacles than for neighboring targets. However, the post-hoc paired sample t-tests (see Appendix B, Table B19) revealed that only the comparison between the two Types of Neighbor in the BOTH condition $t(11)$ = 4.28, p = .001 was significant, while the other differences were not big enough to withstand the correction of alpha after Bonferroni (α = 0.05/9 ≈ 0.006). Hence, the effect of the Type of Neighbor only matters crucially, when subjects did both tasks at once. For non-significant results of paired sample t-tests, see Appendix B, Table B19.

The interaction effects between Task and Type of Fixated Object ($F(2,22)$ = 0.10, p = .902), between Type of Fixated Object and Type of Neighbor ($F(1,11)$ = 3.04, p = .109) or the 3-way interaction ($F(2,22)$ = 0.75, p = .486) were not found in the present data (see Appendix B, Tables B10 and B20 to B22).

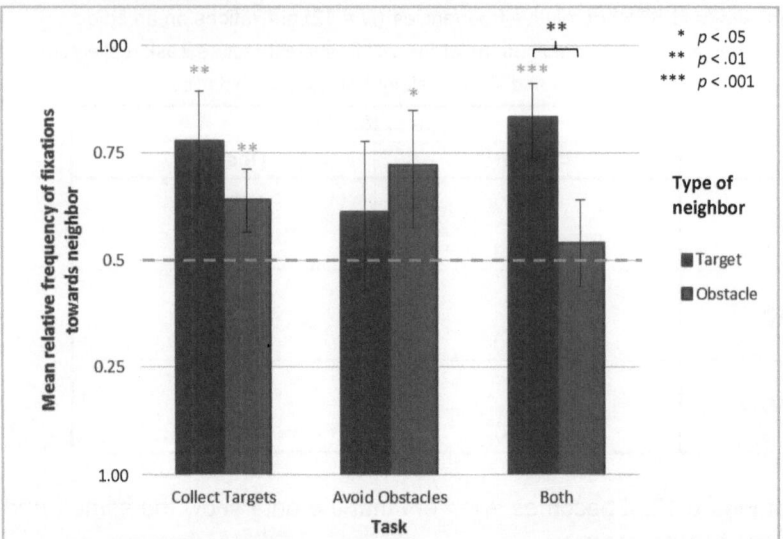

Figure 13. The means of relative frequencies (N = 12) of fixations on an object biased towards a neighbor for the three different Tasks (collect targets vs. avoid obstacles vs. both at once) and the different Types of Neighbor (target vs. obstacle). For details on figure elements, see Figure 8; black stars mark results of post-hoc comparisons via paired sample t-test (α adjusted after Bonferroni: α per test = 0.05/9 ≈ 0.006).

3.3. Screening of Possibly Interfering Direction Effects

Since the total number of fixations in each bin varied dramatically between and within subjects (see Appendix B, Table B2), it is possible that the effects described above are a consequence of two mostly independent direction effects: a direction preference of gaze (left vs. right) and a higher number of neighboring objects to one side than to the other (left vs. right) due to mere object configuration. Assuming, for instance, a 100% gaze preference to the left while there were only situations with neighbors on the left side of the fixated object, one can see easily that the resulting gaze bias *towards* neighbors would be entirely ascribable to the coincidence of the former two.

Because the dependent variable in the previous analysis of variance was computed by the relative direction of gaze and the relative direction of the neighbor (see section 3.2.1. The Computation of a New Variable), a mediator analysis with these two factors would explain the variance in the dependent variable thoroughly. For this reason, two further analyses of variance were conducted to examine if those two kinds of direction effects were present in the data.

3.3.1. Direction Preferences of Gaze

As before, a 3-way analysis of variance (ANOVA) was conducted for the three within-subject factors Task (CT, AO, BOTH), Type of Fixated Object (target, obstacle) and Type of Neighbor (target, obstacle; see Appendix B, Table B23). This time, the dependent variable was the *gaze position relative to the center of the fixated object* (left vs. right of center; see Figure 6B). Again, paired samples *t*-tests have been conducted post-hoc to further compare significant effects; to examine if the relative frequencies for fixations in a certain direction were different from chance, one sample *t*-tests have been computed. The critical alpha level was set to 5% for all analyses with a Bonferroni adjustment for the paired sample post-hoc *t*-tests.

The ANOVA revealed a significant main effect for the Type of Fixated Object, $F(1,11) = 9.03$, $p = .012$ (see Appendix B, Table B24). The obtained means are displayed in Figure 14 ($M_{Targ} = 0.352$, $SEM_{Targ} = 0.035$; $M_{Obst} = 0.493$, $SEM_{Obst} = 0.054$; see Appendix B, Table B25). The one sample *t*-test, became significant for fixated targets only ($t_{Targ}(11) = -4.05$, $p = .002$; $t_{Obst}(11) = -0.14$, $p = .893$; see Appendix B, Table B26). Taken together, these results point to a gaze bias with a preference to the left side of the object center, but only if the fixated object was a target.

71

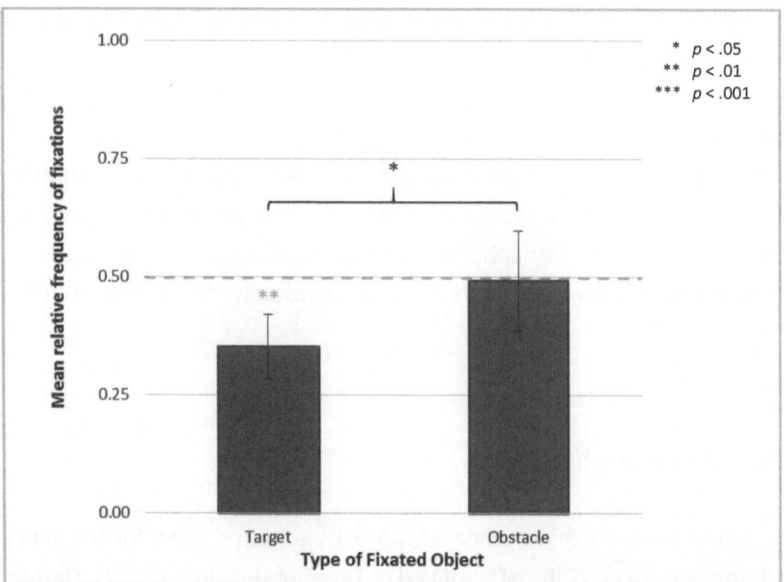

Figure 14. The means of relative frequencies (N = 12) of fixations on an object biased towards the right side of the object for the different Types of Fixated Object (target vs. obstacle). Values above chance (dashed line) indicate a more frequent occurrence of fixations biased to the *right*; values below indicate a more frequent occurrence of fixations biased to the *left* side. Grey stars mark results of one sample t-tests against chance; black stars mark results of the 3-way ANOVA. Error bars represent the confidence interval of 95%.

Additionally, a significant interaction between Type of Fixated Object and Type of Neighbor, $F(1,11)$ = 11.79, p = .006 (see Appendix B,Tables B24 and B27 to B29), was obtained, whereas no other effect reached a significant level in the ANOVA (see Appendix B, Table B24). Neither the Type of Neighbor, nor the Task, taken by themselves, had significant impacts on the data, $F_{Nb}(1,11)$ = 0.62, p =.449; $F_{Task}(2,22)$ = 0.27, p = .768 (see Appendix B, Tables B30 and B31). The same held true for the interaction between Type of Fixated Object and Task, $F(2,22)$ = 0.96, p = .399 (see Appendix B, Table B32), the interaction between Type of Neighbor and Task, $F(2,22)$ = 0.31, p = .632 (adjusted after Greenhouse-

Geisser, see Appendix B, Tables B33 and B34), and the 3-way interaction, $F(2,22) = 0.14$, $p = .873$ (see Appendix B, Table B35).

3.3.2. Differences in the Configuration of Objects

Once again, a 3-way analysis of variance was conducted for the three within-subject factors Task (CT, AO, BOTH), Type of Fixated Object (target, obstacle), and Type of Neighbor (target, obstacle; see Appendix B, Table B36). Here, the *position of the neighboring object relative to the fixated object* (left vs. right; see Figure 6C) was set as dependent variable. Importantly, in this particular part of the analysis, no behavioral measure was looked at. The purpose of this analysis was to see, if situations with neighbors on the right or on the left were more likely to occur during the experiment.

Under given sphericity (see Appendix B, Table B37), the ANOVA revealed neither a significant main effect for the different Tasks, $F(2,22) = 0.04$, $p = .960$ (see Appendix B, Table B38), nor for the different Types of Neighbor, $F(1,11) = 4.83$, $p = .0.50$ (see Appendix B, Table B39). Although the latter was close to significance with means of $M = 0.403$ ($SEM = 0.052$) for neighboring targets and $M = 0.255$ ($SEM = 0.029$) for neighboring obstacles (see Appendix B, Table B40). These non-significant results indicate that even though there were differences in object configurations between tasks and between situations with a neighboring target or a neighboring obstacle, they are negligible since they could be due to chance.   .

Yet, there were significant effects for the Type of Fixated Object, $F(1,11) = 5.51$, $p = .039$ and its interaction with the different types of the neighbor, $F(1,11) = 11.96$, $p = .005$ (see Appendix B, Table B39). The first becomes obvious in Figure 15. For fixated targets ($M = 0.266$, $SEM = 0.031$) and fixated obstacles ($M = 0.390$, $SEM = 0.041$) neighbors happened to be more often on their left sides, $t_{FixTarg}(11) = -7.01$, $p < .001$ and $t_{FixObst}(11) = -2.64$, $p = .023$, while this situation seems to be more likely for fixated targets (see Appendix B, Tables B41 and B42).

For details on the interaction effect between Type of Fixated Object and Type of Neighbor, see Appendix Tables B43 to B45.

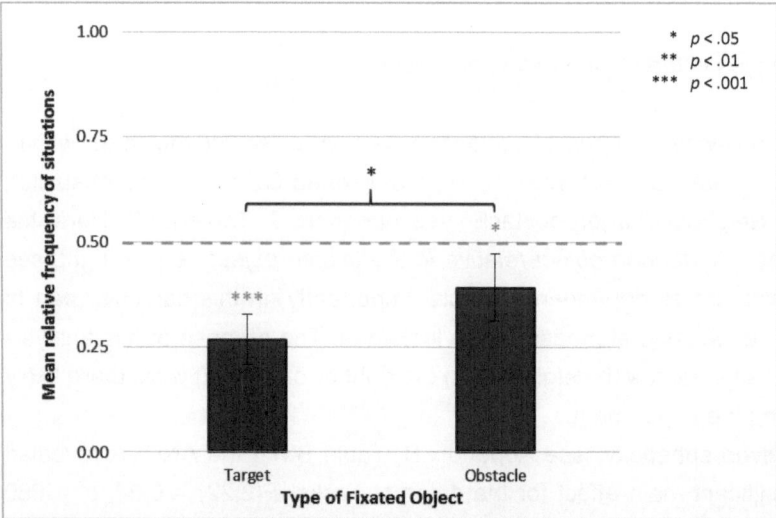

Figure 15. The means of relative frequencies (N = 12) of situations, in which a neighbor was visible in the periphery on the right side of the fixated object, for the different Types of Fixated Object (target vs. obstacle). Values above chance (dashed line) indicate a more frequent occurrence of situations, in which the neighbor was on the *right* side, values below indicate a more frequent occurrence of situations, in which the neighbor was on the *left* side. For details on figure elements, see Figure 14.

The interaction between the Type of Fixated Object and Task, $F(2,22)$ = 3.60, p = .070 (p adjusted after Greenhouse-Geisser; see Appendix B, Tables B37 and B46), as well as the interaction between the Type of Neighbor and Task, $F(2,22)$ = 0.91, p = .418, and the 3-way interaction, $F(2,22)$ = 0.46, p = .639, did not manifest differences in object configurations (see Appendix B, Tables B39, B47 and B48).

3.3.3. Direction Preferences of Gaze for One Visual Object

Another approach to rule out possible effects of a general preferred gaze direction is to consider gaze patterns in situations in which only *one* object is visible. Since there are no other visible objects, a tendency towards one side or the other is thought to be caused by some kind of internal preference. If no such preference is measurable in the one-object situations, it can be assumed that there is no general direction preference when more objects are visible either.

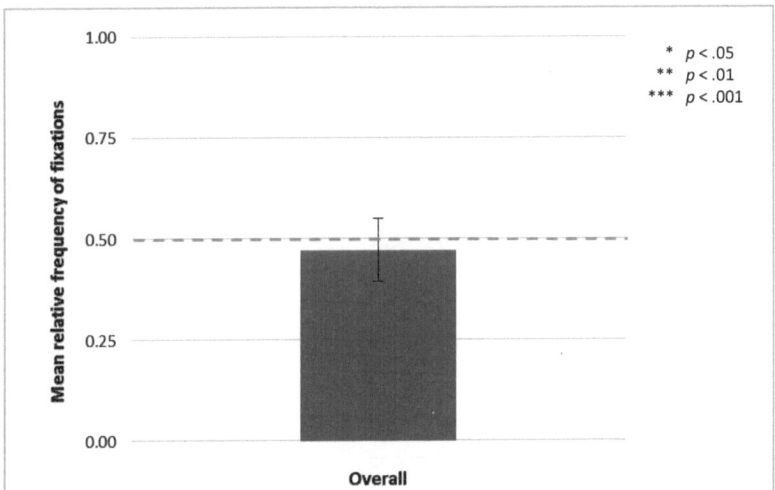

Figure 16. The overall mean of relative frequencies of fixations on the right side of the only visible object in the visual field (averaged across 12 subjects, tasks and object types). Values above chance (dashed line) indicate a more frequent occurrence of fixations biased to the *right;*, values below indicate a more frequent occurrence of fixations biased to the *left* side of the object. Grey stars mark results of one sample *t*-tests against chance. Error bars represent the confidence interval of 95%.

Again, a *t*-test was computed, which tested if the overall mean (averaged across subjects, tasks and object types) of arcsine transformed relative frequencies of fixations on the right side of the one visible object was different from chance. Figure 16 (showing the re-transformed relative frequencies) depicts the overall mean $M = 0.473$ ($SEM = 0.040$) being below chance, which means that a gaze tendency to the left was obtained (see Appendix B, Table B49). However, the t-test was not statistically different from chance, $t(11) = -0.68$, $p = .509$ (see Appendix B, Table B50), that is, there was no crucial direction preference of gaze.

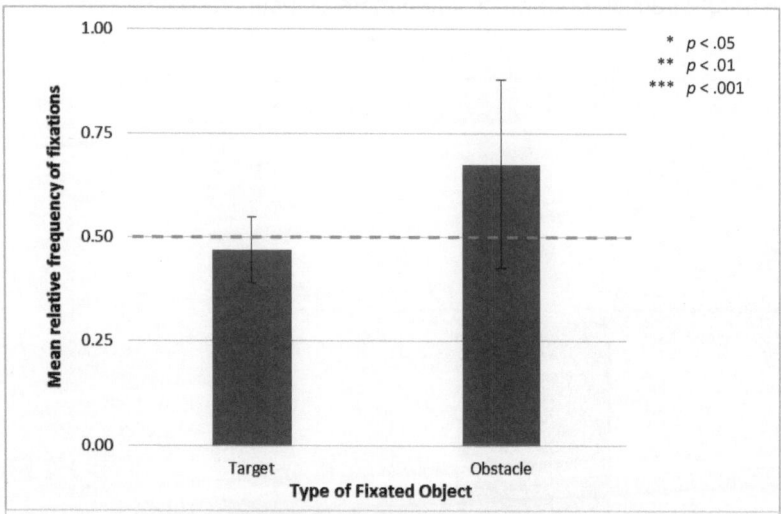

Figure 17. The mean of relative frequencies of fixations on the right side of the only visible object in the visual field for the two different object types (averaged across 12 subjects and tasks). For details on figure elements see Figure 16; α was adjusted after Bonferroni (0.05/2 = 0.025).

Separated by the type of visible object (see Figure 17), subjects seemed to have a preference to the left side when fixating targets, $M = 0.469$ ($SEM = 0.040$) while seeming to prefer the right side of obstacles, $M = 0.674$ ($SEM = 0.116$). Nevertheless, both t-tests did not reveal significant results, $t_{Targ}(11) = -0.78$, $p = .452$ and $t_{Obst}(11) = 1.38$, $p = .196$ (α adjusted after Bonferroni: 0.05/2 = 0.025), which shows again that the differences were trivial (see Appendix B, Table B51 and B52).

In the subsequent chapter 4. *Discussion*, all results presented here will be considered in the broader context of the theoretical background described in section 1. *Introduction*.

4. Discussion

The following sections will discuss the present findings in the framework of bottom-up and top-down theories after summarizing the most important results.

4.1. Summary of Results

In sum, the data revealed that when fixating one of two objects currently present in the visual field subjects allocated their gaze more often towards one side of the fixated object, namely, in the same direction in which the second object was located. In other words, subjects' gaze was biased more frequently *towards* the neighboring object than in the opposite direction. That is, subjects were fixating on the right side of an object center when another object was visible on the right side; respectively, the same was true for the left side. Therefore, the first hypothesis that current information from the peripheral visual field influences gaze position can be corroborated: the gaze bias towards peripheral objects was measurable and significant in this VR experiment.

Furthermore, the interaction between Task and Type of Neighbor, which constituted the task-relevance of the neighboring object, influenced subjects' gazes as well. As stated by the second hypothesis, the general gaze bias towards neighbors (first hypothesis) should be modulated by the current task. More specifically, the gaze bias towards peripheral objects should appear more frequently when these objects are relevant to the current task than when they are not. The results are in line with this statement: As expected, when collecting targets or avoiding obstacles task gaze was clearly biased towards the neighboring object when the neighbor was task-relevant (that is a target neighbor in CT and an obstacle neighbor in AO). In addition, the same effect could be observed for target neighbors when subjects did both tasks simultaneously.

However, several findings of the present study are not in accordance with the second hypothesis. In the collecting targets task, both target and obstacle neighbors produced gaze biases different from chance (as expected by first hypothesis), but their effects did not differ significantly from each other as expected due to task-relevance (second hypothesis). The latter was true in the avoiding obstacles task as well. Here, the gaze bias towards obstacle neighbors should have been more frequent than towards target neighbors due to task-relevance, but again the difference is not statistically meaningful. Moreover, in the avoiding obstacles task, the gaze bias towards neighboring targets was not different from chance in contrast to the prediction of the first hypothesis.

The only task condition, in which a significant difference between target and obstacle neighbors in the frequency of gaze bias was found, was the BOTH task. Admittedly, this result was not expected specifically since both kinds of objects were relevant in this task, however, it is not completely contradictory (for a more detailed discussion, see section 4.3.2. The Task-Relevance of the Neighboring Object). By further looking at the results in the BOTH condition it becomes apparent that the gaze bias towards obstacle neighbors did not occur significantly more frequently than chance. This was somewhat surprising, since it should have been occurred more frequently than chance due to the general bias on the one hand and the task-relevance of obstacles in this task on the other hand.

The post-hoc analyses further revealed that there was no substantial difference between tasks for neither targets nor obstacles. Due to task-relevance, it was expected that these comparisons should show a more frequent gaze bias towards targets in CT and BOTH than in AO and a more frequent gaze bias towards obstacles in AO and BOTH than in CT.

For the comparisons between target neighbors in CT versus BOTH and between obstacle neighbors in AO versus BOTH, no specific results were hypothesized. Two considerations are plausible here: there should either be no difference in the frequency of gaze bias since the objects are relevant in both tasks. Alternatively, the gaze bias frequency should be reduced in the BOTH condition, since here attention is spread to more than one task at a time.

Although these results are partly incompatible with the a priori hypotheses, the data pattern, even though *not* significant, showed the expected tendency in some cases: in CT, the tendency to direct gaze in the direction of a neighboring target happened more frequently than when the neighbor was an obstacle. The expected opposite was true for AO: the gaze bias towards obstacle neighbors was more frequent than for target neighbors. Furthermore, the gaze bias towards neighboring targets happened more often in CT than in AO and vice versa for obstacles. Plus, as the first hypothesis suggested, the relative frequencies of gaze bias for neighboring targets in AO and neighboring obstacles in BOTH were higher than chance – that is, a gaze bias towards the particular neighbor, albeit not significant.

It is also important to mention that the effects described so far do not seem to trace back on any kind of a general direction preference. If there had been a bias to either the right or the left without any neighbors that could have attracted gaze, then it would have had to be assumed that such a direction preference also occurs in situations with more than one present object and that this in turn influences the results for the gaze bias towards neighbors. This can be ruled out since no such gaze direction preference was found in situations in which only one object, either target or obstacle, was present in the visual field. Hence, the gaze bias towards neighbors is no artifact of other effects.

In this regard, it is important to point out, that there has been a significant gaze preference effect due to the Type of Fixated Object in cases of two visible objects (see section 3.3.1. Direction Preferences of Gaze). That is, when targets were fixated, gaze was directed more often to the left than to the right side of the object center. Since an effect of the Type of Fixated Object was not expected for the gaze bias towards the neighbor, this direction preference when fixating targets is not problematic for the interpretation. If anything, it is helpful to explain the unexpected main effect of Type of Fixated Object for the gaze bias towards neighbors (see section 3.2.2. The Analysis of the Gaze Bias Towards Neighboring Objects). The results show that fixations were biased more often towards the neighbor than away from it only when a target was fixated. This unexpected effect can be affiliated to the coincidence of (a) the gaze preference effect to the left when fixating targets and (b) the fact that in these situations neighbors were more frequently visible on the left side of the fixated target (see section 3.3.2. Differences in the Configuration of Objects).

Further intriguing findings, although not expected, were the differences in *total* numbers of fixations due to the Type of Fixated Object and the current Task. In general, subjects made considerably less fixations upon obstacles than on targets, independent of their task-relevance. Additionally, the total number of fixations in the AO task was much less than in CT and BOTH. Hence, although these two factors had no noteworthy effects on the investigated gaze bias, still, they seem to influence subjects' gaze behavior as indicated by the differences in total numbers (see section 4.3.1. The Task-Relevance of the Fixated Object).

After having summarized the most important results, the next section will interrelate the present findings to previous results in the framework of bottom-up processes.

4.2. A Visual Center of Gravity Effect in Real-Life Tasks

The results revealed that when two objects were present in the subject's visual field and one of the objects was fixated that subject's gaze was biased more often towards the second object than away from it. This was demonstrated for almost all object configurations: Significant biases were found for neighbors on the left and on the right side of the fixated object, for fixated targets, and for target and obstacle neighbors. The only analysis that could not reach statistical significance was the one for fixated obstacles. However, even in this case the expected tendency was obvious in the data. The non-significance can be ascribed to the very small number of fixations on obstacles and the ensuing lack of power (see section 3. Results).

These results go hand-in-hand with several findings on the visual COG effect described above (see section 1.4.3. Findings on the Visual Center of Gravity Effect). Although the present study did not quantify the strength or the spatial extent of the visual COG effect, it does constitute a first attempt to verify the existence of a more or less bottom-up driven gaze bias towards objects other than the currently fixated one, using VR (for the top-down interpretation see section 4.3. The Task-Relevance of Objects and its Impact on Gaze Position). That is why, next, the present results will be related to previous COG results and ideas for further investigation will be given.

Coren and Hoenig (1972) showed that a visual COG effect occurs when non-task-relevant distractors are presented and that the resulting gaze bias is stronger the more distractors were shown. Since in the present study, a gaze bias towards neighbors independent of their task-relevance (non-relevance corresponds to distractors) was found, the results are conform. Additionally, a similar analysis of the impact of the neighbor number is also possible for the current data: Are the effects shown here more dominant the more neighbors are visible in the periphery? Is there a positive correlation between the number of objects in the periphery and frequency of the gaze bias? If so, does this relation only work up to a certain number of objects, indicated by an asymptotic approximation in a normally distributed dependent variable? These questions could be addressed by looking at situations in which more than two objects are visible.

Coren and Hoenig (1972) also found that the visual COG effect was stronger when the distractor was presented between the fixation point and the target (see also Findlay, 1982). One interpretation is that eccentricity – in other words the distance from fovea – plays a crucial role and that the influence of peripheral information decreases with increasing eccentricity. To investigate this in the present study the distance between fixated object and neighbor would need to be quantified (see section 4.5. Prospects). Cohen and Hoenig's results suggest that the closer the neighbor to the fixated object the more impact it has on gaze. This hypothesis is limited since it would suggest the greatest impact on gaze when the two objects are right next to each other. This situation does not leave the possibility to let gaze fall between the objects, since there is no space between them anymore. Moreover, this would also contradict their own results showing that the visual COG effect increases with increasing distance between objects. These conflicting predictions are due to different considerations of weights on the visual COG and due to other dependent variables in classical laboratory experiments than in real-life tasks (see section 1.2. A Brief Glance on the Subject of Visual Attention). Nevertheless, it would be an interesting study to determine if either of these two effects can withstand the naturalistic setting.

A further interesting result in the real-life context was pointed out by Findlay (1982). According to his results, the visual COG effect can be influenced by the size of neighbor, namely that saccades are more likely to land closer to the bigger of two objects. In real-life, or respectively, in a VR set-up, the size of an object coincides with the distance between subject and object. To quantify this distance is delicate since the subject is moving. For instance, when the subject is fixating one of two visible objects and at the same time moves towards those objects, then the subject's gaze might be fixed while the images of the objects on the retina increase in size. Therefore, it would be difficult to determine the impact of object size in the course of a fixation. The simplest solution would be to investigate saccadic landing positions because they are not vastly extended over time. To actually examine if object size has a gradually increasing effect on gaze bias, one would need to relate the distance between subject and object to the relative size of the object in the visual scene at – theoretically – any given point in time.

Talking about natural settings, Vishwanath and Kowler (2003 & 2004) already showed that there is a visual COG effect for naturalistic objects, and that the COG is stronger in more than in less naturalistic tasks. This suggests that the visual COG effect can occur in daily life. And that is what can be concluded from the current study as well. A gaze bias, comparable to the visual COG effect, was demonstrated in a life-like VR set-up suggesting that peripheral information impacts gaze.

Unlike other authors (e.g. Zhao, et al., 2012), here, this bias is not interpreted as an error in the calculation of gaze allocation (see section 1.5. The Paradigm and the Aim of the Study): By allocating gaze to intermediate spots rather than to a certain object of interest alone a greater amount of useful information about the current state of the world, is provided. Consequently, this can be a helpful strategy in situations in which the economy of time to derive information is more important than its quality. For instance, it is necessary to gain quick information about the locations of the ball and two opponents as in the illustration at the beginning (see section 1. Introduction). It is important for the goalkeeper to be able to make fast decisions and in turn enact fast reactions. If the outcome, namely the chosen reaction, is reliably successful, then this strategy provides a faster and less expensive alternative to saccadic sequences.

In contrast to this point of view is the assumption of non-compromise gaze according to the authors of the Walter model (Sprague et al., 2007). The effect that gaze allocation is influenced by the existence of objects in the periphery can be interpreted as a compromise in gaze allocation as stated out in the paradigm (see section 1.5. The Paradigm and the Aim of the Study). Instead of making fixations upon one object after another, which would provide highly accurate information – but is rather expensive in terms of economy of time and saccadic initiation – gaze is directed to one object with a bias towards the other to get a higher amount of poorer quality information in shorter time. Thus, there actually seems to be compromises in gaze allocation in natural tasks that can serve more than one visual operation. Sprague et al. (2007) argued that this is unlikely for reasons of too little incremental information. However, as pointed out, the findings here tell another story. They contradict this basic assumption of the Walter model that every fixation can only serve one task at a time (Sprague et al., 2007).

The following suggestions shall resolve this contradiction. A new parameter should be added to the arbitration level of the model allowing Walter's fovea to make compromises between several tasks, that is, making fixations to positions that serve more than one currently active task. This does not mean that this is the best strategy to reduce uncertainty and maximize reward in every situation, task, or context. However, it is another possibility to enhance predictions of human behavior. By allowing compromises in gaze, uncertainty is reduced in more than one microbehavior, which can be advantageous in terms of gaining reward. Of course, peripheral information is not perfect due to decreasing accuracy, and using it for updating the microbehaviors about the current state might therefore be problematic in certain situations. On the other hand, there might be other situations in which this less reliable information is good enough for the update. For instance, when the task is very simple, not of high priority, or when the information acquiring needs to be prompt, this strategy can be useful.

Of course, foveal vision should still be acknowledged as being "special". That is, foveal vision is the main provider of useful information, which enables humans to interact successfully with their environment. Humans are therefore primarily driven by top-down processes to accomplish cognitive or behavioral goals. Still, peripheral vision should not be left unconsidered. To concede at least a minor role to peripheral vision as suggested by the overall gaze bias in the present data, a certain amount of systematic bias towards peripheral objects should be added to Sprague et al.'s algorithm. This should shift Walter's gaze, as predicted by reward and uncertainty, towards the visual COG of the currently visual scene. Further experiments will be necessary to examine if the new parameter improves the predictions for human behavior in a significant way that would justify the consideration of a further parameter.

Up to this point, the interaction effect of Task and Type of Neighbor, that is the task-relevance of the neighbor, has not been reflected. The next section will concern this topic in terms of previous findings and the suggested Walter add-on.

4.3. The Task-Relevance of Objects and its Impact on Gaze Position

This section deals with the relevance of the objects in the currently running task and how this factor can influence gaze allocation. Therefore, it is subdivided into two units. The first part will be about the task relevance of the fixated object (see section 4.3.1. The Task-Relevance of the Fixated Object), while the second will discuss the task-relevance of non-fixated neighboring objects (4.3.2. The Task-Relevance of the Neighboring Object).

4.3.1. The Task-Relevance of the Fixated Object

As known from a wide variety of previous studies, the relevance of objects in the current task influences gaze (Rothkopf et al., 2007; Shinoda, et al., 2001; Sullivan et al., 2012; Tong & Hayhoe, 2014), that is for instance, objects are fixated more frequently when they are task relevant. In the present study, the equivalent of the task-relevance of the fixated object was the interaction of Task (CT, AO, BOTH) and the Type of Fixated Object (target, obstacle). Here, this effect did not produce significant differences in the frequency of the gaze bias towards neighbors. This can be explained by the nature of the dependent variable used here. The better comparison to these previous findings can be made by reviewing the absolute numbers of fixations in Tables 1 to 4. They reveal a data pattern – although not tested on significance – as suggested by previous studies: In the CT and BOTH tasks, the proportion of fixations towards targets (task-relevant) is highest, whereas this number drops in AO, in which targets are not task-relevant. In turn, in AO the highest number of fixations on obstacles (task-relevant) can be seen in comparison to the other two tasks. This is somehow surprising since obstacles are also task-relevant in the BOTH condition. Another contradictive result is that even in AO the number of target fixations (not task-relevant) was higher than the number of obstacle fixations (task-relevant). For possible explanations of the latter, see section 4.4. *Alternative Explanations and Limitations of the Study*.

After this brief consideration of the task-relevance of the fixated object, the task-relevance of the neighbor will be discussed more comprehensively in the following.

4.3.2. The Task-Relevance of the Neighboring Object

As shown in the present study, task relevance of the neighbor (i.e. the interaction between Task [CT, AO, BOTH] and Type of Neighbor [target, obstacle]) has an influence on the gaze bias. More specifically, peripheral information seems to be taken more into account when currently important for the task. This suggests that

87

the COG-like bias found here, which from the perspective of visual COG literature is mainly bottom-up driven, can be influenced by top-down processes as the current behavioral goal.

Another top-down influence was shown by Coëffé and O'Regan (1987), in whose experiment the predictability of target location affected the visual COG effect. The possibility to influence the visual COG effect, in turn suggests, that this phenomenon can be a helpful, at least partly top-down driven, strategy rather than being an error (see section 1.5. The Paradigm and the Aim of the Study). If it were an error, the task-relevance of the neighboring object would not produce differences in the gaze bias. Since an influence of the neighbor's task-relevance was found here, it supports the idea of this gaze bias as potentially useful alternative in gaze allocation strategies (see section 4.2. A Visual Center of Gravity Effect in Real-Life Tasks).

The data pattern revealed herein did not exactly mirror the predicted results (see section 4.1. Summary of Results). Mainly, it was unexpected that the results of the post-hoc *t*-tests only revealed a significant difference between targets and obstacles in the BOTH condition, but not in CT or AO. Since targets are task-relevant in CT and obstacles are task-relevant in AO, it was expected to find a significantly higher frequency of gaze bias towards task-relevant neighbors than towards non-relevant neighbors in CT and AO as well.

Besides the lack of power due to small numbers of fixations (see section 4.4. Alternative Explanations and Limitations of the Study), there are two obvious possibilities that might have produced this data pattern. The first possible explanation is an effect of task order. Since the BOTH condition was always the last block for each subject, they might have had developed certain strategies in the two preceding blocks and somehow combined them in the third block, which resulted in the difference.

The second possibility goes hand in hand with the new parameter suggested in section 4.2. *A Visual Center of Gravity Effect in Real-Life Tasks*, but needs an additional expansion of the Walter model. To lead to this further add-on, the assumed underlying mechanisms need to be declared at first.

It is conceivable, that the difference in the *number* of relevant tasks produces the data pattern. According to the data, the relevance of the neighbor is only of importance when *two* tasks need to be done at once. In the single task conditions (CT and AO), it is *either* collecting targets *or* avoiding obstacles, in other words one after another, whereas in the BOTH task the subjects had to make sure to avoid the obstacles *while* collecting the targets. Based on this premise, the obvious preference for neighboring targets over neighboring obstacles in the BOTH condition can be explained by the different qualities of implicit reward gained from the two different tasks. When targets are collected, a desired positive consequence is obtained, which in terms of operant conditioning (Skinner, 1938) works as a positive reinforcement. This implicit positive consequence is indicated by the cheerful fanfare sound that is played when subject successfully collect a target.

On the other hand, when avoiding obstacles the inner drive to accomplish the task derives from the avoidance of negative consequences, that is the concept of punishment according to Skinner (1938). Whenever the subject failed to successfully avoid an obstacle, the subject was "punished" by an annoying buzzer sound.

Positive reinforcement results in an enhancement of desirable behavior, here, collecting the targets, while punishment results in a decrease of undesirable behavior, here, making contact with obstacles. Therefore, the latter are avoided. Both, positive reinforcement and punishment result in accomplishing the corresponding task. Still, differences due to the underlying mechanisms of the two are conceivable.

Since these assumptions are reasonable in the framework of reward learning, it would be sensible to draft another add-on to the Walter model to see, if it would further enhance its predictions. This second add-on would need to modulate the first gaze bias parameter (see section 4.2. A Visual Center of Gravity Effect in Real-Life Tasks). Namely, in such a way that in cases of multiple running tasks, the systematic gaze bias towards neighbors is varied by quality of reward. That is, a higher prioritization parameter would need to be assigned to positive reinforced tasks like CT than to penalized tasks such as AO.

It needs to be emphasized again, that these changes are only *suggestions* derived from the present study. Of course, the present findings should first be replicated and further examined to rule out alternative explanations and improve some shortcomings, each of which will be the topics of the next section.

4.4. Alternative Explanations and Limitations of the Study

Several aspects of this study have to be viewed in a critical light and due to methodical constraints and compromises in the analyses, the results presented here are quite limited.

One of the main aspects contributing to the limitations of the conclusions above is the small number of actual analyzed fixations (see section 3.1. Total Frequencies of Fixations and Exclusion of Data). On average only 64 fixations per subject were analyzed (see Appendix, Table B1). Especially the number of fixations on obstacles (about one sixth of fixations on targets) and the number of fixations in the AO task were extremely small. The small number of fixations on obstacles is a possible account of why the gaze bias towards neighbors is not statistically different from chance for fixated obstacles; it is likely that it is due to a lack of power. However, the question is: how can this "preference" for targets be explained?

Several answers are conceivable. First, this result might have occurred simply due to the nature of the two different tasks. Targets are unavoidable since they have to be gathered by walking through them. Thus, approaching the target leads to a relative enlargement of the target in the visual field, so that the subject has no other choice than to look at it. Obstacles might not necessarily be fixated since subjects avoid getting too close to them (Rothkopf et al., 2007).

Second, the small number of fixations on obstacles might be due to subjects' memorization of the object configuration when looking at the path at the beginning of the trial. However, this seems unlikely for different reasons: first, the total number of objects along the path varied between 6 and 14. Although it seems possible to remember the location of six objects (for limitations of visual working memory, see section 1.3.1.2. Composition of Behavior), it is quite impossible for more objects even if intended. Additionally, since all objects were on each subject's individual eye height, some objects are covered by others and are not visible at once.

Third, the minority of fixations on obstacles might be able to shed further light on human gaze strategies. Since the total numbers of fixations for each possible combination of factors were not balanced, they were not independent from subjects' behavior. Explicitly, subjects "decided" – more or less intentionally – where they looked. Based on this premise, one can argue that the difference pointed out by the first line of reasoning (see above) is not due to different strategies subjects have to use, but rather those they are able to use appropriately in the corresponding situation. That is to say, targets are fixated with the intention to collect them. Obstacles, on the other hand, might not need to be fixated since it is more important to guide one's way *around them* as people do every day. By reviewing the video sequences, it became apparent that subjects often looked right next to an obstacle, which is assumed to be the way they were planning to take for passing the obstacle without making contact. Thus, it seemed like the information of the actual positions of obstacles is not essential for the avoidance, so that there is less need to employ foveal vision for its provision. Information about the obstacles position provided by peripheral vision seemed to be sufficient for this navigating task and targets seemed to be "more important" to employ foveal acuity for.

This goes along, at least partly, with the findings of Rothkopf et al. (2007) showing that the distributions of gaze locations were different between targets and obstacles: Targets were primarily fixated at their centers, whereas obstacles were primarily fixated at their edges (see Figure 6 in Rothkopf et al., 2007). If the criteria of the fixation finder algorithm had been adjusted in the present study, particularly, if the size of the 'virtual fovea' were bigger, probably more fixations that were close to the objects would have been labeled as 'on object'. This can explain why Rothkopf et al. found fixations on obstacles edges, while here fixations on obstacles were quite rare.

However, about 29% of missing values have been substituted by chance in the preparation for the analyses (see section 3.2.2. The Analysis of the Gaze Bias Towards Neighboring Objects), which was reasonably conservative since it counteracted the statistical significance of effects. Admittedly, in terms of inferential statistics it would have been superior to balance the number of situations across tasks and object types. However, as pointed out above, this way, it was possible to get an impression of where subjects decided to look.

Despite this conservative procedure, some statistically significant and intriguing effects were revealed, hence, they seem fairly robust (also shown by mainly small SEM) and are thought to be easily replicable.

After having discussed the missing values, another aspect that needs to be reviewed critically is that there was no center category in the present study. As a result, the relative fixation positions were labeled either left or right of the object center, no matter the distance of the fixation position from the object center. What if a center category, that is virtually a 'no effect detectable' category, had been considered? Fixations close to the center would not have been counted as left or right, or respectively in advanced analyses as same or opposite, but rather as 'not affected by peripheral information'. It is necessary to allow this additional categorization to make sure that the effect is strong enough to withstand it, but this is an issue of future analysis using a metric dependent variable (see section 4.5. Prospects). Notwithstanding, reviewing the video sequences showed that gaze position was clearly divergent from the object center in most cases.

A further point of criticism is that while examining the influence of peripheral objects, the possible impact of objects in the background (e.g. desks, shelves, and doors) or the elevator were not considered in the analysis. Rothkopf et al. (2007) showed that fixation time spent on objects in the background in a virtual walking paradigm is negligible. Of course, effects of peripheral information about these objects cannot be ruled out; however, since they were not task-relevant and held constant in each room, their effect is assumed to be negligible here as well. More critical is the disavowal of the elevators. The green elevator disk is at least partly task-relevant in terms of staying on the path and take the elevator to the next floor to end the current trial. The reason why the elevator was not considered here was that it has not been viewed as being *primarily* relevant like the more demanding tasks of collecting targets or avoiding obstacles.

In the context of not considering peripheral objects, another shortage is worth mentioning. Because only the movements of the subjects' left eye were tracked and the video sequences only showed what the left eye was seeing, everything that was visible on the further right side of the subject's visual field (i.e. information provided by the right eye) was not open to scrutiny. Thus, objects on the right side might have influenced gaze as well but could not be considered since they were not objectively visible.

Up to this point, the present findings were related to previous results and theories, a new parameter for the Walter model was suggested, shortcomings in the procedure were revealed and ideas on alternative explanations and future investigations were presented. The next section will give an overview about reasonable prospects in the near future.

4.5. Prospects

So far, relative frequencies of fixations biased towards neighbors were presented as a first hint on possible effects of peripheral information on gaze in VR set-ups. Since the extent of the effect is not deducible yet, a reasonable next step is to quantify the effects above. Explicitly, investigating if and how peripheral information influences gaze position, using a metric rather than a dichotomous variable (same vs. opposite) used here. One possibility for such a metric variable is the relative distance between gaze position and the object center (see bottom part of Figure 18). Thereby it is possible to get an indirect estimate of the peripheral information used to plan eye movements and to get an idea of the bias' magnitude. Moreover, it would be possible to compare the data to the results of Rothkopf et al. (2007) on differences in gaze distribution.

Additionally, when using a metric variable a center category will be necessary to see, if the gaze bias towards neighbors can withstand a consideration of a category declared as 'no effect of peripheral information on gaze' (see section 4.4. Alternative Explanations and Limitations of the Study).

In a further step, a quantification of the relative positions of neighbors can be implemented and interrelated to the first variable (see black lines in Figure 18). Thereby, it would be made possible to estimate the impact of neighbors according to their distance to the fixated object.

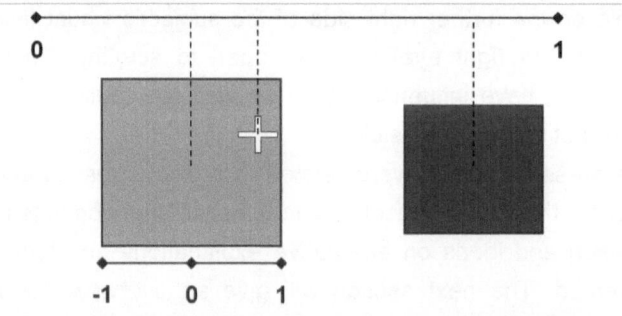

Figure 18. An illustration of the quantification of positions and distances between objects and gaze (white cross). The black line on top represents the width of the screen; the black dashed lines the positions on screen. The light grey line at the bottom shows the measurement of distance from gaze position to the object's center. By marking the center of the fixated object (white cube) by 0 and the outer edges by 1 or -1, it is possible to quantify the relative extent of the gaze bias towards the neighbor (grey cube).

In addition, this would allow the examination of fixations *between* objects. By this means, incremental knowledge about the usage of gaze strategies in this paradigm can be provided.

4.6. Conclusion

The goal of the present study was to investigate if information provided by peripheral vision influences the allocation of gaze in a naturalistic task, namely while walking. When fixating an object, subjects' gaze was biased more often *towards* a second object in the periphery than in the opposite direction. This bias could be shown for neighbors on the left and the right side, in all three tasks (collect targets, avoid obstacles or doing both at once), for both types of the neighbor object (target or obstacle), and for fixated targets. This suggests that objects other than the fixated one, in other words, objects perceived by peripheral vision, do indeed influence the position of gaze.

Moreover, an effect of the neighbor's task relevance was revealed, but only when subjects were doing both tasks at the same time. If in further experiments the hypothesized impact of the neighbor's task relevance is not vindicated as well for single tasks, then, the differences found here can be explained in terms of positive reinforcement and punishment producing different results.

Overall, the present results constitute a suggestion that effects of peripheral vision on gaze can be shown in VR set-ups and therefore are believed to occur in daily life.

Additionally, this bias is interpreted as a useful gaze strategy in certain situations rather than being an error in gaze allocation. For this reason, models of human gaze allocation such as the Walter model (Sprague et al., 2007) should consider peripheral information as a further parameter in their algorithms.

5. References

Ballard, D. H., Hayhoe, M. M., & Pelz, J. B. (1995). Memory representations in natural tasks. *Journal of Cognitive Neuroscience, 7*(1), pp. 66-80. doi:10.1162/jocn.1995.7.1.66

Ballard, D. H., Hayhoe, M. M., Pook, P. K., & Rao, R. P. (1997). Deictic codes for the embodiment of cognition. *Behavioural and Brain Sciences, 20*, pp. 723-767. doi:10.1017/S0140525X97001611

Ballard, D. H., Kit, D., Rothkopf, C. A., & Sullivan, B. T. (2013). A hierarchical modular architecture for embodied cognition. *Multisensory Research, 26*, pp. 177-204. doi:10.1163/22134808-00002414

Brooks, R. A. (1986). A robust layered control system for a mobile robot. *IEEE Journal of Robotics and Automation, 2*, pp. 14-23. doi:10.1109/JRA.1986.1087032

Clark, A. (1999). An embodied cognitive science? *Trends in Cognitive Sciences, 3*, pp. 345-351. doi:10.1016/s1364-6613(99)01361-3

Coëffé, C., & O'Regan, J. K. (1987). Reducing the influence of non-target stimuli on saccade accuracy: Predictability and latency effects. *Vision Research, 27*(2), pp. 227-240. doi:10.1016/0042-6989(87)90185-4

Coren, S., & Hoenig, P. (1972). Effect of non-target stimuli upon length of voluntary saccades. *Perceptual and Motor Skills, 34*, pp. 499-508. doi:10.2466/pms.1972.34.2.499

Diaz, G., Cooper, J., Rothkopf, C., & Hayhoe, M. M. (2013). Saccades to future ball location reveal memory-based prediction in a virtual-reality interception task. *Journal of Vision, 13*(1), pp. 1-14. doi:10.1167/13.1.20

Engbert, R., & Kliegl, R. (2003). Microsaccades uncover the orientation of covert attention. *Vision Research, 43*, pp. 1035-1045. doi:10.1016/S0042-6989(03)00084-1

Encyclopaedia Britannica (2014). Keyword: *"Centre of Gravity"*. Retrieved June 03, 2014, from http://www.britannica.com/EBchecked/topic/242556/centre-of-gravity.

Ernst, M. O., & Bülthoff, H. H. (2004). Merging the senses into a robust percept. *Trends in Cognitive Sciences, 8*(4), pp. 162-169. doi:10.1016/j.tics.2004.02.002

Findlay, J. M. (1982). Global visual processing for saccadic eye movements. *Vision Research, 22,* pp. 1033-1045. doi:10.1016/0042-6989(82)90040-2

Firby, R. J., Kahn, R. E., Prokopowicz, P. N., & Swain, M. J. (1995). An architecture for vision and action. *Proceedings of the 14th International Joint Conference on Artificial Intelligence, 1,* pp.72-79.

Gegenfurtner, K. R. (2006). *Gehirn & Wahrnehmung* (4. ed.). Frankfurt a. M.: Fischer Taschenbuch Verlag.

Goldstein, E. B. (2008). *Wahrnehmungspsychologie - Der Grundkurs.* (H. Irtel, Ed., & G. Plata, Trans.) Berlin, Heidelberg: Spektrum Akademischer Verlag.

Guez, J.-E., Marchal, P., Le Gargasson, J.-F., Grall, Y., & O'Regan, J. K. (1994). Eye fixations near corners: Evidence for a center of gravity calculation based on contrast, rather than luminance or curvature. *Vision Research, 34*(12), pp. 1625-1635. doi:10.1016/0042-6989(94)90122-8

Hafed, Z. M., & Clark, J. J. (2002). Microsaccades as an overt measure of covert attention shifts. *Vision Research, 42,* pp. 2533-2545. doi:10.1016/S0042-6989(02)00263-8

Hayhoe, M. M., Shrivastava, A., Mruczek, R., & Pelz, J. B. (2003). Visual memory and motor planning in a natural task. *Journal of Vision, 3,* pp. 49-63. doi:10:1167/3.1.6

Henderson, J. M., Pollatsek, A., & Rayner, K. (1989). Covert visual attention and extrafoveal information use during object identification. *Perception & Psychophysics, 45*(3), pp. 196-208. doi:10.3758/BF03210697

Hess, R. F., & Holliday, I. E. (1992). The coding of spatial position by the human visual system: Effects of spatial scale and contrast. *Vision Research, 32*(6), pp. 1085-1097. doi:10.1016/0042-6989(92)90009-8

Hirsch, J., & Mjolsness, E. (1992). A center-of-mass computation describes the precision of random dot displacement discrimination. *Vision Research, 32*(2), pp. 335-346. doi:10.1016/0042-6989(92)90143-7

Hoffman, J. E., & Subramaniam, B. (1995). The role of visual attention in saccadic eye movements. *Perception & Psychophysics, 57*(6), pp. 787-795. doi:10.3758/BF03206794

Irtel, H. (2013). *Experimentalpsycholoisches Praktikum - Nachdruck für das Experimentalpsychologische Praktikum der Justus-Liebig Universität Giessen* (2. ed.). Berlin, Heidelberg, New York: Springer-Verlag.

Itti, L., & Koch, C. (2000). A saliency-based search mechanism for overt and covert shifts of visual attention. *Vision Research, 40*, pp. 1489-1506. doi:10.1016/S0042-6989(99)00163-7

Kolb, B., & Whishaw, I. Q. (1996). *Neuropsychologie* (2. ed.). (M. Pritzel, Ed., M. Mauch, M. Niehaus-Osterloh, & M. Numberger, Trans.) Heidelberg, Berlin, Oxford: Spektrum Akademischer Verlag.

Kolb, B., & Whishaw, I. Q. (2001). *An Introduction to Brain and Behaviour.* New York: Worth.

Land, M., Mennie, N., & Rusted, J. (1999). The roles of vision and eye movements in the control of activities of daily living. *Perception, 28*, pp. 1311-1328. doi:10.1068/p2935

Luck, S. J., & Vogel, E. K. (1997). The capacity of visual working memory for features and conjunctions. *Nature, 390*, pp. 279-281. doi:10.1038/36846

Marr, D. (1982). *Vision - A computational investigation into the human representation and processing of visual information.* San Francisco: W.H. Freeman and Company.

McGowan, J. W., Kowler, E., Sharma, A., & Chubb, C. (1998). Saccadic localization of random dot targets. *Vision Research, 38*(6), pp. 895-909. doi:10.1016/S0042-6989(97)00232-0

Morgan, M. J., Hole, G. J., & Glennerster, A. (1990). Biases and sensitives in geometrical illusions. *Vision Research, 30*(11), pp. 1793-1810. doi:10.1016/0042-6989(90)90160-M

Nave, C. R. (2012). Keyword: "Center of Mass". *Hyperphysics.* Retrieved June 03, 2014, from http://hyperphysics.phy-astr.gsu.edu/hbase/cm.html

Neider, M. B., & Zelinsky, G. J. (2006). Scene context guides eye movements during visual search. *Vision research, 46*(5), pp. 614-621. doi:10.1016/j.visres.2005.08.025

Pinel, J. P. (2009). *Biopsychology* (7. ed.). Boston: Allyn and Bacon.

Posner, M. I. (1980). Orienting of attention. *Quarterly Journal of Experimental Psychology, 1*, pp. 3-25. doi:10.1080/00335558008248231

Rothkopf, C. A., & Ballard, D. H. (2013). Modular inverse reinforcement learning for visomotor behaviour. *Biological Cybernetics, 107*, pp. 477-490. doi:10.1007/s00422-013-0562-6

Rothkopf, C. A., Ballard, D. H., & Hayhoe, M. M. (2007). Task and context determine where you look. *Journal of Vision, 7*(14), pp. 1-20. doi:10.1167/7.14.16

Schneider, W. X., & Deubel, H. (1995). Visual attention and saccadic eye movements: Evidence for obligatory and selective spatial coupling. In J. M. Findlay, R. Walker, & R. W. Kentridge, *Eye movement research - Mechanisms, processes and applications* (pp. 317-324). doi:10.1016/S0926-907X(05)80027-3

Schütz, A. C., Trommershäuser, J., & Gegenfurtner, K. R. (2012). Dynamic integration of information about salience and value for saccadic eye movements. *Proceedings of the National Academy of Sciences, 109*(19), pp. 7547-7552. doi:10.1073/pnas.1115638109

Shinoda, H., Hayhoe, M. M., & Shrivastava, A. (2001). What controls attention in natural environments? *Vision Research, 41*, pp. 3535-3545. doi:10.1016/S0042-6989(01)00199-7

Skinner, B. F. (1938). *The Behavior of Organisms: An Experimental Analysis*. New York: Appleton-Century-Crofts.

Sprague, N., Ballard, D. H., & Robinson, A. (2007). Modeling Embodied Visual Behaviours. *ACM Transactions on Applied Perception, 4*, pp. 1-25. doi:10.1145/1265957.1265960

Stritzke, M., Trommershäuser, J., & Gegenfurtner, K. R. (2009). Effects of salience and reward information during saccadic decisions under risk. *Journal of the Optical Society of America, 26*(11), pp. 1-13. doi:10.1364/JOSAA.26.0000B1

Sullivan, B. T., Johnson, L., Rothkopf, C. A., Ballard, D. H., & Hayhoe, M. M. (2012). The role of uncertainty and reward on eye movements in a virtual driving task. *Journal of Vision, 12*(13), pp. 1-17. doi: 10.1167/12.13.19

Tong, M. H., & Hayhoe, M. M. (2014). The effects of task and uncertainty on gaze while walking. *Poster presentation at NETI 2014 at The University of Texas at Austin.*

Triesch, J., Ballard, D. H., Hayhoe, M. M., & Sullivan, B. T. (2003). What you see is what you need. *Journal of Vision, 3,* pp. 86-94. doi:10:1167/3.1.9

Vishwanath, D., & Kowler, E. (2003). Localizaion of shapes: eye movements and perception compared. *Vision Research, 43,* pp. 1637-1653. doi:10.1016/S0042-6989(03)00168-8

Vishwanath, D., & Kowler, E. (2004). Saccadic localization in the presence of cues to three-dimensional shape. *Journal of Vision, 4,* pp. 445-458. doi:10.1167/4.6.4

Vitu, F. (1991). The existence of a center of gravity effect during reading. *Vision Research, 31,* pp. 1289-1313. doi:10.1016/0042-6989(91)90052-7

Wandell, B. A. (1995). *Foundations of vision.* Sunderland, Massachusetts: Sinauer Associates.

Whitaker, D., McGraw, P. V., Pacey, I., & Barrett, B. T. (1996). Centroid analysis predicts visual localization of first- and second-order stimuli. *Vision Research, 36*(18), pp. 2957-2970. doi:10.1016/0042-6989(96)00031-4

Wyszecki, G., & Stiles, W. S. (2000). *Color Science: Concepts and Methods, Quantitative Data and Formulae* (2. ed.). New York: John Wiley & Sons.

Zhao, M., Gersch, T. M., Schnitzer, B. S., Dosher, B. A., & Kowler, E. (2012). Eye movements and attention: The role of pre-saccadic shifts of attention in perception, memory and the control of saccades. *Vision Research, 74,* pp. 40-60.doi:10.1016/j.visres.2012.06.017